EATING DISORDERS:
DECODE THE CONTROLLED CHAOS

YOUR KNOWLEDGE MAY JUST SAVE A LIFE

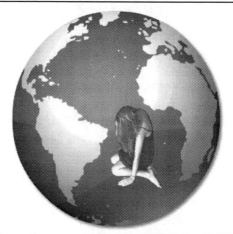

Erica Ives, M.A., MFT, CEDS
Marriage and Family Therapist
Certified Eating Disorder Specialist

BALBOA
PRESS
A DIVISION OF HAY HOUSE

ISBN: 978-1-4525-4826-5 (sc)
ISBN: 978-1-4525-4825-8 (e)

Library of Congress Control Number: 2012906817

Balboa Press books may be ordered through booksellers or by contacting:

Balboa Press
A Division of Hay House
1663 Liberty Drive
Bloomington, IN 47403
www.balboapress.com
1-(877) 407-4847

Because of the dynamic nature of the Internet, any web addresses or links contained in this book may have changed since publication and may no longer be valid. The views expressed in this work are solely those of the author and do not necessarily reflect the views of the publisher, and the publisher hereby disclaims any responsibility for them.

The author of this book does not dispense medical advice or prescribe the use of any technique as a form of treatment for physical, emotional, or medical problems without the advice of a physician, either directly or indirectly. The intent of the author is only to offer information of a general nature to help you in your quest for emotional and spiritual well-being. In the event you use any of the information in this book for yourself, which is your constitutional right, the author and the publisher assume no responsibility for your actions.

Printed in the United States of America

Balboa Press rev. date: 3/14/2013

This book is written through my eyes, my soul, my heart, my mind, and my body, accompanied by the shared experiences of so many others, who have traveled on the path of recovery from an imprisoning eating disorder. My goal in writing this book is to help ensure that others TAKE NOTICE of these silent screams for help. I have touched the tears, seen the utter despair, heard the whispers of hell, and witnessed death within the realm of this disease. I have also held the hands of hope and courage, witnessed growth through trust and renewed faith, and seen others choose to live instead of simply exist. We need to open our eyes, we need to pay more attention, and choose to intervene. So, if I can reach one person who is willing to take extra notice then we have quite possibly saved a life.

Contents

PREFACE

Eating Disorders have a tremendous effect on the quality of life, and impact all levels of functioning. More often than not, however, there is a tendency to turn a blind eye to this deadly disease. By reading Decode the Controlled Chaos, one will gain knowledge about the diagnostic criteria utilized to classify different types of eating disorders, to instruct in the detection of early warning signs and symptoms, and to provide an understanding of the serious medical complications that can arise as a result of an active eating disorder. In addition, this book explains the importance of treatment using a multi-disciplinary team approach, identifies the "Level of Care" guidelines for patients suffering from eating disorders, and the most successful treatment options and protocols.

─── 1 ───

ALL ABOUT EATING DISORDERS

What is an Eating Disorder?

We cover up our wounds with healing ointment and gauze in an attempt to heal ourselves, but despite our efforts, an emptiness wells up inside. We try to fill this emptiness with food, self-destructive behaviors, and activities, but what we really yearn for is wholeness.

-Harville Hendrix

Eating disorders such as *Anorexia, Bulimia, Binge Eating Disorder,* and *Eating Disorders Not Otherwise Specified* are marked by severe and extreme disturbances in eating behaviors, related thoughts, and emotions. They are insidious, imprisoning, and pervasive. Eating disorders permeate all aspects of a sufferer's life, and have profound effects on the individual who is suffering and that individual's loved ones. Once "it" has its grip on oneself or a loved one, the sun stops shining and the flowers stop blooming. The eating disorder becomes the only thing that matters. Eating disorders do not discriminate; they are found in every culture, religion, ethnicity, and socio-economic group.

Eating disorders are extremes in eating behaviors - a diet that never ends. Eating disorders involve intense preoccupation with behaviors and rituals surrounding food. Some examples include obsessively counting calories, binging on food in secret, throwing up after eating, and following rigid diets. However, while eating disorders may begin with a preoccupation with food, shape, and weight, they are about much more than food. People with eating disorders usually use food and the control of food in an attempt to compensate for emotions that may otherwise seem too overwhelming.

Eating disorders serve as an attempt to adapt and cope in a world in which the sufferer feels completely unequipped to navigate. This could cause anyone to feel out of control. The sufferer seeks control through food, but the truth of the matter is that the food is actually controlling them, and they are therefore, "losing control." An eating disorder can also serve as an adaptive function by providing comfort in a world where the sufferer feels alone, unsupported, invalidated, and possibly unloved. The eating disorder can provide friendship, companionship, support, validation, and even love. This may seem an odd concept, but by reading further you will gain a further glimpse into the world of eating disorders.

Another adaptive function eating disorders may serve is as a distraction from the difficulties of life. The sufferer may feel overwhelmed by the responsibilities and demands of everyday life. They may lack a strong sense of self or identity. They have learned to shut down, shut out, disconnect, run away, avoid any possible perceived threat of abandonment, unpredictability, being too much or not enough, being smothered, controlled, or ignored, or any number of seemingly dangerous turns in the road. The eating disorder can provide an "alter" identity or its very opposite, a way to disappear. Either way, it serves as a way to cope with life.

Eating disorders can also serve as a way to communicate. They speak the unspoken. Every eating disorder has a voice, a story, and a thought, a feeling that the sufferer is trying to express. The deeper the sufferer has fallen into the grips of an eating disorder, the more disconnected they become from their voice, their story, their thoughts, and their feelings. The eating disorder speaks what one is truly missing and seeking in life. The sufferer is seeking comfort and safety from pain, to be understood, to feel worthy and accepted, an identity, and approval. They are seeking hope and relief from their inner confusion and turmoil.

Eating disorders affect individuals on a physical, emotional, cognitive, interpersonal, and spiritual level. The body begins to deteriorate, the senses become dulled, the ability to think clearly and rationally becomes impaired, cognitive processing actively slows, and access to one's emotions diminishes. Depression and anxiety lead to isolation and exhaustion. These effects then set in even deeper, and the closest of relationships become less of a priority. Eating disorder sufferers focus all of their energy and attention into the dark world of their eating disorder, often leaving their family, loved ones, and friends behind. Eating disorder sufferers believe they have literally become their eating disorder. They are unable to decipher any separateness from the disorder that has become their sole identity. This all results in a complete disconnect from human experiences such as love, gratitude, honesty, compassion, and feeling a sense of life with meaning and purpose.[83]

How do we characterize an eating disorder? At the very least, it is a scary, dark, secretive, lonely existence that is often glorified and pursued. Through the use of food and a complete preoccupation with weight, shape, and appearance, sufferers use eating disorders as a way of trying to make sense of a world that otherwise feels senseless, to feel hope in a world that feels hopeless, to feel successful in a world where sufferers believe they are never enough or simply too much. An eating disorder becomes an eating disorder, of course when all of the diagnostic criteria are met. Beyond the diagnostic criteria, when the eating disorder becomes the sole way of expressing what one believes cannot be expressed in any other way, it is most definitely time to reach out for help.

An eating disorder...when have I ever really not had an eating disorder. This craziness became my identity when I was just a child, a little girl. Actually, I don't really remember much of my life without my eating disorder. I never felt like I fit in, not even at home- the place I would imagine I should feel the safest, whatever that really means. I just know I felt sad, lonely, and worried more often than not. I especially worried about my family. Maybe my mom told me, maybe she didn't, but somehow I knew how to care for them, watch out for them, and even protect them. I don't think anyone was really doing those things for me, but the message was that I am the stronger one, the more responsible one, and the more rationale one. So, the message was to stay in control, don't fall apart, don't cause problems, and in fact don't let anyone see your weaknesses. BE IN CONTROL! So, I did what I thought I was told. I was the good girl, I kept things in control, everything from my room, my closet, my emotions, my food, my routine, my exercise, my thoughts. As much control as I thought I had, the world inside and outside of me felt crazy, scary and dark. I was screaming and crying inside but I did everything I could to turn it all off. While I thought I had CONTROL over my food, my weight, and my body, the CHAOS that was in my head NEVER stopped. This is the meaning of controlled chaos.

Causes and Risk Factors of Eating Disorders

Your present circumstances don't determine where you can go; they merely determine where you start.

-Nio Dubei

There is no single cause of eating disorders. They are complex illnesses with numerous contributing factors. They arise from interplay of psychological, emotional, interpersonal, biological, social and cultural factors. No one factor means that someone will develop an eating disorder. Scientists and researchers are still learning about the underlying causes of these damaging disorders.

Case vignette of interplay of factors:

Marie, a 25-year-old woman who has struggled with anorexia for the past ten years remembers her problems with her relationship with food beginning as early as she can remember. Her parents were divorced when she was five. She also has two siblings, a younger sister and older brother. Her father basically abandoned his children. Her mother was a hard worker and dedicated mother. Even as a single mother, she worked on her Master's degree, worked full time with no additional financial help, always picked up her children at the end of their school day and had dinner on the table every evening. Marie's mother was also quite preoccupied with appearance and mastered every new diet that came on the market. Marie somehow connected to her mother's struggles. She began to feel different than other kids at a very young age. Marie called sick from school quite frequently because she wanted to be with her mother. She helped out however she could and helped care for her younger sister who was much more "dramatic and emotional." Marie did not do this because she was directly asked to by her mother; it was just an unspoken role she took on. Marie disconnected from her emotions at a young age. Her perfectionistic traits were seen early on as well. She would spend hours in her sketching beautiful women in beautiful gowns. She also had a dollhouse that became her fantasy world. Every room was decorated to the tee. Marie never explored make up and is an absolutely beautiful girl. She reached puberty later than the other girls, between 15-16 years old, and expressed discomfort with her emerging femininity. Food and exercise became her sources to try and make sense of the world around her. She had an early understanding that if she did not eat as much food there would be enough for everyone else. She once expressed that she does not want or feel deserving of taking up too much space. Then she became an avid runner. She ran a 5 and 10k on a weekly basis. She described her running as a just a way to try to "run" away from it all. She continued to suffer in silence. The story continues with the development of the food rituals and the rigidity of her routine. But she had already turned off her voice, disconnected herself so profoundly from her truths to simply survive in her world.

Psychological and Emotional Factors

There are many psychological factors that contribute to an eating disorder. A common thread among all eating disorders is low self-esteem.[92] Self-esteem is the degree to which an individual values and respects him or herself, and is proud of his or her accomplishments. According to Steinhausen (1993), characteristic components of low self-esteem are insecurity, negative mood and depression, poor body image, feelings of inadequacy, social and personal withdrawal, poor adaptation skills, and unrealistically high aspirations. All of these traits are seen fairly consistently in individuals suffering from eating disorders. Research indicates that there are certain genetic psychological traits, known as vulnerability traits that predispose certain individuals to the development of eating disorders. These include personality traits such as perfectionism, obsession, and/or anxiety. In addition, there is often a high level of emotional vulnerability within those who develop eating disorders.

Emotional vulnerability is defined by these characteristics:

• Very high sensitivity to emotional stimuli,

• Very intense response to emotional stimuli, and

• A slow return to an emotional baseline once emotional arousal has occurred.[57] This is most likely due to a combination of biological predisposition, and environment.

The way in which an individual deals with their emotions may also be a contributing factor to the development of an eating disorder. Impairment of the ability to identify an emotional state accurately, to express emotions safely, and to adjust or regulate internal experiences is most often a contributing factor to the development of eating disorders. Emotional regulation refers to a person's ability to be aware of, identify, understand and accept his or her emotional experience and to engage in behaviors to manage uncomfortable emotions. People with good emotion regulation skills are able to control the urges to engage in impulsive behaviors during times of emotional stress. They are also able to soothe themselves in a way that allows them to refocus attention back on rational thinking and/or the task at hand without staying completely immersed in their emotional state. Someone who develops an eating disorder most likely has deficits in these areas. They experience negative emotions more often and more intensely than others and for numerous reasons do not know how to effectively manage their emotions. If an individual has no access to a consistent and coherent framework for interpreting and tolerating emotions, that individual may look to external sources for distraction from distressing emotions.

Interpersonal Factors

It is important to explore the role that relationships, with family and peers, contribute to the onset of eating disorders. Rather than blame, it is about possible environmental and interpersonal factors that can put one at a greater risk for the development of an eating disorder. Interpersonal experiences that have most frequently linked to the development of eating disorders include abuse, trauma, and teasing.

The manner in which an individual perceives and then internalizes the experiences and relationships with others differs from person to person. Therefore, the child who has poor emotional regulation skills or the inherent personality traits noted earlier (i.e., perfectionism, obsessive, anxiety, or heightened sensitivity), is more likely to perceive, experience, and internalize particular family relationships and dynamics in an extremely harmful way.

Family Relationships

Family relationships are complex, and are central to the development of a child's sense of self. This early caregiving relationship has a profound effect on the child's ability to deal with adversity. Parents are not taught how to parent differently based on the uniqueness of each child; therefore, it is also important to note that while a particular parenting style may be successful with one child, it may have negative effects with another child. However, the predisposition of a particular child contributes to the outcome no matter what the type of parenting style.

Researchers have found several "typical" family types and there has been much focus on the development of healthy emotional boundaries in families. In some cases, families are over-involved and enmeshment with a parent may develop. "Enmeshed" is a psychological term describing a symbiotic and overly intimate relationship in which the emotional and psychological boundaries between two people have become so obscure or unclear, that it is difficult for the two to function as separate individuals with their own identities. Varying degrees and intensity of "enmeshment" or "over-involvement" are apparent within what are considered to be healthy families, especially between mothers and daughters. Since enmeshment represents a continuum, the extent of a negative impact on the child will vary. However, when there are conflictual effects of enmeshment, they most often emerge during adolescence. It is during this developmental period that the adolescent is increasing independence and identity outside of the family and ultimately striving for healthy differentiation.

Differentiation is described as the capacity of the individual to function autonomously, making self directed choices, while remaining emotionally connected to the intensity of a significant relationship system.[51] This means learning how to function as an individual within the family group. If this developmental task is met with resistance from a parent, the child may attempt to ignore the desire to be independent in order to avoid conflict and disappointment. In order to develop a separate identity from the over-involved parent, the adolescent may try to exert independence and autonomy through a relationship with food and the body.

An "invalidating" environment in the home refers to a failure to treat an individual in a manner that conveys attention, respect, and understanding. Invalidation may lead to confusion about all aspects of self. When a child's thoughts or feelings are dismissed or minimized, criticized, teased, or judged on an excessively frequent basis, food may easily become that external source that successfully distracts from the feelings the child would rather avoid. Additional examples of an invalidating family environment include not being taken seriously, being disregarded by family, finding a lack of support for the development of the authentic self, being treated unequally with respect to another sibling. Invalidation may also result in the inability to trust one's own experience within self and the outside world. This lack of trust of self, others, and the world at large, may manifest itself as a lack of trust in one's own body, relationship with food, and a preoccupation with weight, shape, and appearance.

Research also indicates that families of individuals with eating disorders tend to be overprotective, perfectionistic, rigid, and focused on success. They have high, sometimes unreasonable expectations for achievement and may place heightened attention on external rewards. Many children from these kinds of families try to achieve the appearance of success by being thin and attractive. If a child perceives that they are failing to live up to family expectations, they may turn to something that seems more easily controlled and at which they may be more successful, such as food restriction or weight loss. Familial characteristics of women with eating disorders may also include a family environment in which discussion of weight and appearance are common.[40] Research also suggests that daughters of mothers who have a history of eating disorders may be at higher risk for developing an eating disorder. These factors indicate that some of the thoughts and behaviors of eating disorders may be learned through parental modeling.

All families have their areas of dysfunction, some more severe than others. Some individuals who develop eating disorders live in or came from families that exhibited negative behaviors, such as alcohol or drug use. Marital discord, divorce, and even domestic violence are other family issues often associated with an eating disorder. However, family dysfunction, and every family has some, does not necessarily equate to the development of an eating disorder.

1. *The first time when I was 14 years old, I already knew by then that I hated my body. I was always the chubby one; my sister was the skinny perfect one. My mom let me know that part of being pretty is being thin, but I liked to eat. It made me feel good or at least better. Looking back I realize that sometimes I ate out of boredom, sometimes just because I could, often when I was angry, frustrated or uncomfortable. But, I wasn't aware of my emotions during that time. I remember my family dinners. I ate as quickly as I could and usually more than anyone else. But, I remember watching my sister, who picked and picked at her food. I started to get stomachaches during dinner and excuse myself to use the bathroom. This began to happen more frequently. My mother never confronted me because I would respond in anger or simply know how to convince her how physically horrible I felt that she would then focus only on what she could do to make me feel better. I was seen as the volatile child. My mom did not want to upset me because she was afraid of how I would act out, and I believe her denial was how she tried to protect herself. I was so consumed with my own thoughts that I truly didn't even care how she felt.*

2. *I am now 22 years old and I remember growing up in pretty "normal family." My parents are still married, I attended private school, and I always had nice clothes. But what I did see in my home, was a mother who herself was consumed with body appearance and dieting. She was also very*

self-critical. My mother believed that happiness came from the outside in versus from the inside out. I definitely internalized this belief that my mother carried. The message of to be lovable you must be thin. To be happy you must be thin. As much as my mother told me I was beautiful, the "not quite good enough though...." was communicated through very mixed messages.

Peer Relationships

With regards to peer relationships, especially during the teen years, it is common for youth to seek acceptance from one another. There is so much pressure for teens to fit in and feel like they belong. Adolescents are trying to become comfortable with their bodies and all of the many physical and emotional changes they are experiencing.

Puberty poses a particular risk for the development of eating disorders, especially among girls. Puberty is the most common period for onset of eating disorders, such as bulimia nervosa (BN), with onset of binge-eating peaking at 16 years and the onset of purging at 18 years.[18] Puberty among females is accompanied by weight gain from fat tissue, which is considered by many girls to be undesirable.[37,100] The bodily changes inherent in puberty, and their implications, may also contribute to an eating disorder in a child who is not emotionally and physically ready to grow up. If a child develops sooner than others, if they are teased or ridiculed based on size, weight, or a physical flaw, if they are more introverted or shy, or is seen above average intelligence by their peers, this can lead to both depression and obsessive weight concerns and body-image issues. An individual may use food and the control of food as an attempt to deal with or avoid feelings that may otherwise seem overwhelming.

Life Transitions

Life transitions can cause heightened emotional distress, which could cause one to be more susceptible to developing an eating disorder. Some examples of life transitions include leaving home for college, a major move, an illness, pregnancy or the beginning or break up of a relationship. Other risk factors include living in a sorority house, involvement in athletics, and being in an occupation that focuses on weight. The impact of stressful life events is at least partially dependent upon how individuals perceive, or think about these experiences, and how they attempt to cope with them. Even though these life transitions are normative, this does not mean that have the same affects on all individuals.

When Jennifer, age 18, first appeared at her university's mental health clinic for intake, she appeared to be much like her fellow freshmen. Eager, alert, and challenging, she gravitated to a prelaw curriculum. But, unlike her peers, from the first week of school, Jennifer was also completely preoccupied with food. In her dormitory, it seemed as though food was everywhere. Away from home for the first time, she could now eat as she wished and do as she wished. Shocked and dismayed by the degree of anxiety she experienced in her solitude, Jennifer sensed that college would be a greater challenge for her than she had ever thought. She had not anticipated her reaction to loneliness and to the intense competition of her peers.

Sexual Abuse

There is a strong correlation between sexual abuse and eating disorders. The presence of sexual abuse among women is of an epidemic proportion, with prevalence estimates of lifetime sexual abuse varying between 15 and 25% among the general female population.[19] The strongest association between sexual abuse and eating disorders has been found among individuals with bulimia. When combined with other psychiatric co-morbidity, particularly substance abuse, bulimia has been linked with higher frequency and more severe history of sexual abuse.[19]

Many have described the act of purging as a way to discard or rid the self of "dirty" guilty and shameful feelings, as well as intrusive thoughts and memories that may be a direct result of sexual abuse. The effects of abuse are commonly manifested as a disgust towards one's body, as the trauma has occurred directly to the mind and body. Whatever type of abuse has occurred (physical, emotional, or sexual), the relationship to the body may become filled with fear, mistrust, confusion, and a sense of powerlessness. Children may learn to blame themselves to think that everything is their fault, that they cannot do anything right, that that they are not deserving of love. Moreover, some victims of sexual trauma may wish to be thinner, to minimize secondary sex characteristics, and to appear less attractive to potential perpetrators.[64] Both researchers and clinicians agree that traumas resulting from a history of sexual abuse are contributing factors that can play a role in severe body image disturbance and the development of an eating disorder.

How could someone have done this to me? How could someone I trusted have done this to me? I hate that I kept this secret for so long. But I was scared: scared that no one would believe me, terrified that it was my fault, my fault for letting this happen. I hated my body. I despised everything about my body. I hated feeling anything in my body. I loathed feeling hunger pains and I especially detested feeling full and everything in between. I wanted to be empty because I felt gross and dirty most of the time. So, sometimes I went for days without eating but then it was just too much and I ate. But, I ate and ate until I was so full that I felt even more disgusting and repulsed. As if that was even possible...I had to get rid of that food inside me and I would go to whatever means possible. I would throw up until I felt empty and numb again. Then I was so tired that I just wanted to go to sleep. But then I woke up and I felt guilty and ashamed. The only thing that would make the guilt and the shame go away was when I was successful in depriving myself of food or getting rid of all of it inside of me.

Biological/Genetic Factors

Scientists are still researching possible biological and genetic causes of eating disorders. Within the past decade there has been a dramatic increase in research funding to investigate the specific genetic basis of eating disorders.

Researchers have identified specific chromosomes that may be associated with bulimia and anorexia. In particular, regions on chromosome 10 have been linked to bulimia as well as obesity. Some evidence has reported an association with genetic factors responsible for serotonin, the brain chemical involved with both well-being and appetite. Researchers have also identified certain proteins that may influence an individual's vulnerability to developing an eating disorder.

Family and twin studies suggest a strong genetic component in the development of anorexia and bulimia nervosa, but the specifics of exactly what vulnerabilities are transferred and the mechanisms by which they contribute to the pathogenesis of eating disorders need to be identified. Genetics research and investigations into hormonal and neurotransmittal links are the most frequently explored areas of biological explanations for eating disorders; research into hereditary personality types is also being conducted.[93] Dr. Thomas R. Insel, M.D., Director of the National Institute of Mental Health, in an October 5, 2006,[45] letter to the Chief Executive Officer of the National Eating Disorders Association stated the following:

"Research tells us that anorexia nervosa is a brain disease with severe metabolic effects on the entire body. While the symptoms are behavioral; this illness has a biological core, with genetic components, changes in brain activity, and neural pathways currently under study."

There is increasing evidence that anorexia nervosa is associated with abnormality in neural circuits that modulate aspects of emotion and cognitive control.[71] Anorexic individuals tend to be over-controlled and rigid, and they exhibit personality characteristics such as low impulsivity and high harm avoidance. These features are consistent with the formulation or anorexia nervosa as a neurobiologically-based disorder that is characterized by accentuated inhibition and control[98] and may be due to fundamental alterations in the neurobiological control mechanisms that govern behavior, emotion and physiology.[20,49,71]

In some individuals with eating disorders, certain chemicals in the brain that control hunger, appetite, and digestion have been found to be unbalanced. The exact meaning and implications of these imbalances continues to remain under investigation.

Social and Cultural Factors

Warning-reflections in this mirror may be distorted by socially constructed ideas of beauty.

-Anonymous

A widely held theory indicates that poor body image, which may lead to the development of eating disorders, is in part caused by a culture that values appearance over internal essence and values women more when they are thin. Body image refers to one's own personal perception of one's physical appearance based on self-observation and the subjective reactions of others. Body image affects how one thinks and feels about oneself as a person. This image is not based on facts, it is personal perception, in other words on one's psychological image of oneself. Therefore, poor body image results not only in being dissatisfied and unhappy with one's body, but also in, believing others' perceptions are the same. It is important to recognize that in learning to be women in our society, we have accepted, and even internalized, what is all too often a derogatory and constraining image of ourselves[85] can lead eventually to poor body image and eventual development of eating pathology.

Mass media has immense power to reinforce the development of poor body image and that can result in deadly eating disorders. The media responds to the cultural and economic drive for thinness, and also feeds the obesity epidemic. Images of the "perfect" or "ideal" female body are everywhere. Celebrities are consistently becoming younger and thinner. On the other hand, the media floods the public with ads promoting the consumption of unhealthy foods and poor eating habits. Media can also give children and teens contradictory messages about dietary habits and ideal body type

Media advertising on media such as magazines, television, and the Internet are sending very dangerous images and messages, which contribute to further to poor body image. You have seen it, "I've lost 20 lbs. on this diet and I can finally put on my size 2 jeans again- I feel great," she says provocatively staring into the eyes vulnerable women. Then you hear the messages on the radio and it goes something like this, "Ladies, are you constantly trying to lose that extra 10-20 lbs. in your mid section that won't go away no matter what you do. Well our product promises this result and all you need to do is call for a free trial." Media advertising even goes so far to place these commercials on the channels that children watch. Then there is the advertising in magazines where the front cover either criticizes the celebrity who has gained a few pounds or praises the actress who is withering down to nothing. The advertiser then, in such a subtle manner, places these photos side by side for even a greater impact. Media and advertising sells so much more than products; the media sells values, unrealistic expectations, and ideals of success and self-worth. Body image distortion for young women begins to grow through comparison with unrealistic body images and the creation of unrealistic expectations of the self. Poor body image has the potential to grow into an eating disorder as media advertising draws the person in ever deeper. Even more, media does not teach individuals how to listen their bodies, value their own unique internal experience, or how to accept the diverse differences in natural body sizes. Instead our culture's ideals and media advertising increases the pressure to become thinner, more perfect, and to conform to one ideal. Losing 10 lbs., going to the gym five days a week, limiting daily caloric intake to a specific number no longer seems to be enough. There becomes a very vicious cycle and a recipe for disaster: this continual striving for perfection and control that never seems achievable, or enough.

By choosing to remain unaware of the deep seriousness of this ever-present influence, the repetitive message and the subliminal impact of advertising, we ignore one of the most powerful "educational" forces in our culture. It is important to emphasize that these advertising images and messages do not cause the eating disorder, but they are a large contributing factor to what shapes one's body image. Although the cultural demands placed upon the body may change over time, these spoken and unspoken cues that come through all these channels continue to have a huge impact on an individual's self-esteem and sense of well being.

Co-morbid Conditions and Eating Disorders

Eating disorders have substantial co-morbidity (more than one psychiatric disorder) with other psychiatric disorders and conditions, including mood disorders, anxiety disorders, substance use disorders, and personality disorders.[44] Due to the nature and focus of this book, this section provides limited information on the diagnoses outside of eating disorders. These diagnoses are not to be taken lightly and require the appropriate professionals to make the determination if the diagnosis is indeed present, and if so, how best to proceed with treatment.

The Diagnostic and Statical Manual of Mental disorders provides a definition of each mental disorder, a common language, and standard criteria for the classification of the mental disorders, some which are listed below. However, it is important to note that the DSM-IV-TR, soon to be *DSM-5, is a very complicated manual and was created for and used by numerous treatment professionals. To elaborate a bit further, some of these terms you have and are about to learn are listed throughout this section. The DSM-IV-TR organizes each psychiatric diagnoses into five dimensions (axes) relating to different aspects of each disorders. Listed below are the five axes along with some examples of each category:

Axis I refers to Clinical Disorders and some of these include eating disorders, all mood disorders, and anxiety disorders including post-traumatic stress disorder.

Axis II excludes all diagnostic categories except Mental Retardation and Personality Disorders. Some examples of Personality Disorders include borderline personality disorder, obsessive-compulsive personality disorder, narcissistic personality disorder, and histrionic, avoidant, and dependent personality disorder. Personality disorders fall into three different clusters or categories:

- *Cluster A which is odd or eccentric behavior*

- *Cluster B which is defined by dramatic, emotional, or erratic behavior*

- *Cluster C which is comprised of anxious and fearful behavior*

The fifth edition of the APA's Diagnostic and Statistical Manual of Mental Disorders (DSM-5), set for release in May, 2013, is a manual which contains descriptions, symptoms, and other criteria for diagnosing mental disorders.

Mood Disorders refer to a category of mental health problems that includes all types of depression and bipolar disorder. There are different types of mood disorders, based on their durations, prevalent features and severity of symptoms. The following are the most common types of mood disorders:

- **Major Depression** includes a depressed or irritable mood and a noticeable decrease in interest or pleasure in usual activities, increase or decrease in appetite, insomnia or increase in sleep, feeling worthless or excessive guilt, difficulty concentrating, feeling worthless, and repeatedly thinking about suicide or death.

- **Dysthymic Disorder (Dysthymia)** is a chronic, low-grade, depressed or irritable mood that has endured for about two years. It is accompanied by certain other symptoms such as increase or decrease in appetite, low self-esteem, fatigue or low energy, insomnia or increase in sleep, feeling hopeless and difficulty in making decisions, or in concentrating. These symptoms are persistent, but less severe.[3]

- **Bipolar Disorder,** which has often been referred to as manic depression, includes periods of depression and mania. One may also experience only mania without any depressive episodes. Some of the common symptoms of bipolar disorder are decreased need for sleep, inflated self-esteem or self-importance, easily distracted, excessive talking, increase in goal oriented activities (sexual, work, social, school) or excessive involvement in potentially risky pleasurable behavior. The symptoms can be severe enough to cause harm to self or others. Such patients may need hospitalization to seek appropriate treatment.

Anxiety Disorders include generalized anxiety disorder, social anxiety, panic disorder, simple phobias, obsessive-compulsive disorder (OCD), and posttraumatic stress disorder (PTSD). The anxiety disorders that are most often accompany eating disorders include:

- **Generalized Anxiety disorder** is diagnosed when a person worries excessively about a variety of everyday problems for at least 6 months.[50]

- **Social Anxiety Disorder,** also called social phobia, is diagnosed when people become overwhelmingly anxious and excessively self-conscious in every social situation. People with social phobia have an intense, persistent, and chronic fear of being watched of being judged by others and of doing things that will embarrass themselves.[69]

- **Panic Disorder** is characterized by sudden attacks of terror, usually accompanied by a pounding heart, sweatiness, weakness, faintness or dizziness. Panic attacks usually produce a sense of unreality, a fear of impending doom, or a fear of losing control.[69]

- **Obsessive-Compulsive Disorder** (OCD) includes persistent upsetting thoughts (obsessions) and the use of rituals (compulsions) to control the anxiety theses thoughts produce.[52]

- **Post-Traumatic Stress Disorder (PTSD)** develops after a terrifying ordeal that involved physical harm or the threat of physical harm.[69]

Personality Disorders are a group of psychiatric conditions in which a person's long-term (chronic) behaviors, emotions, and thoughts are very different from their culture's expectations and cause serious problems with relationships and work.[69] Those who struggle with a personality disorder have severe difficulties with relationships. A personality disorder is a deeply ingrained, inflexible pattern of relating, perceiving, and thinking that is serious enough to cause distress or impaired functioning.

Individuals with eating disorders should routinely be assessed by treatment professionals for concurrent disorders. Sometimes these concurrent disorders will preexist eating disorders. It is of importance for a professional to do a thorough assessment to determine whether the presenting symptoms are manifestations of a prominent *Axis I diagnosis or are related to the eating disorder alone.[107] For instance, one may begin to display a social anxiety as a symptom of the eating disorder.

Major depressive disorder and obsessive compulsive disorder are characterized by alterations in inhibitory control and are both consistently reported in the literature to have high comorbid diagnosis in anorexia nervosa.[71,72] Those suffering from bulimia have high prevalence rates of any affective disorder (75%), major depressive disorder (63%), and anxiety disorders (36%).[87] The majority of bulimic patients report that that the initial presentation of the depression or anxiety disorder occurred prior to the presentation of bulimic symptoms. Lifetime co-occurring major depression or dysthymic disorder has been reported in as many as 50%-75% of patients with anorexia and bulimia nervosa.

Substance use disorders are common among individuals suffering from an eating disorder. The National Center on Addiction and Substance Abuse at Columbia University[100] reported that 30 to 70 percent of bulimics have a substance abuse problem. Between 30 and 50 percent of individuals with bulimia and between 12 and 18 percent of those with anorexia, abuse or are dependent on alcohol or drugs,[4,72,100,103] compared to approximately nine percent in the general population.[73,100] Patients with co-occurring substance abuse and anorexia or bulimia nervosa appear to have more severe

---

* The Diagnostic and Statistical Manual of Mental Disorders, 4th. Edition, a manual created for mental health professionals who make psychiatric diagnoses, uses a multiaxial, five dimensional approach to diagnosing. Axis I disorders include the Clinical Syndromes.

problems with impulsivity in general, including greater risk of shoplifting, suicidal behaviors, self-injurious behaviors, and laxative abuse.

Individuals with anorexia nervosa tend to have higher rates of Cluster C personality disorders, particularly obsessive-compulsive, avoidant, and histrionic traits, whereas normal-weight patients with bulimia nervosa are more likely to display features of Cluster B disorders, particularly impulsive, affective, and narcissistic traits. Most sufferers with eating disorders will meet DSM-IV criteria for at least one personality disorder; be it borderline, histrionic, or obsessive compulsive personality disorders. According to the review of the literature, obsessive-compulsive personality disorder is the most common *Axis II diagnosis in eating disordered individuals with restrictive eating behavior, whereas borderline personality disorder is the most common Axis II diagnosis in those with impulsive eating pathology.[88] However, it is important to note, that if features of these personality disorders are present, it does not necessarily mean that they meet a full Axis I disorder.

Research in this area continues to explore the relationship between eating disorders and all of the above mentioned conditions. In addition, when an eating disorder co-occurs with another mental disorder, the treatment needs to be very individualized. The issue of comorbidity and eating disorders is a crucial issue to continually assess and treat throughout treatment.

Athletes and Eating Disorders

Involvement in recreational sports is extremely beneficial in numerous ways. It can help improve self-esteem, build confidence, positively impact body image, assist in the

---

* The Diagnostic and Statistical Manual of Mental Disorders, 4th. Edition, a manual created for mental health professionals who make psychiatric diagnoses, uses a multiaxial, five dimensional approach to diagnosing. Axis II disorders includes the Developmental Disorders and Personality Disorders.

development of a stronger awareness and appreciation of one's relationship to one's body, and build social skills. Competitive athletics can also offer the same benefits as recreational sports; however, there can also be a much darker and dangerous side in the relation of competitive athletics to the development of eating disorders, or at least disordered eating.

Young athletes, particularly dancers, gymnasts, runners, swimmers, and wrestlers, are especially vulnerable to developing eating disorders. Disordered eating can be encouraged or rewarded with athletes because these sports often involve the practice of weight restriction and specific dietary requirements. The higher the level at which one trains, which continually requires more hours, the more difficult and competitive the sport becomes. The National Eating Disorder Association notes that when the pressures of athletic competition are added to an existing cultural emphasis on thinness, the risks increases for athletes to develop disordered eating which may eventually lead to an eating disorder. To make it even more complicated, well-established eating disorders may go undetected in athletes because they tend to look healthier and stronger.

The teen years constitute a vulnerable developmental period and are accompanied by numerous stressors. When the role of being an athlete is added to the many changes and transitions that occur during these challenging years, unique and extensive pressures are greatly increased. They can inevitably lead to increased, even severe psychological and physical stress, which can place an athlete more at risk for developing an eating disorder. Some external pressures include coaches' requirements and expectations, the athlete's own expectations of self, as well as the parent's expectations. Other vulnerability factors for the student athlete include the increasing demands with balancing school and workout hours, time-management, "fitting in" their meals before, during, and after training, as well as dealing with the performance-affecting changes that accompany puberty. Athletic advancement can often be at the expense of personal development.[77] Peer relationships may become more of a struggle due to the different relationships the athletes have with one another versus their peers in school.

> *Being an athlete was just part of my life. That was how I identified myself,*
>
>> *As a dancer....*
>>
>> *As a swimmer....*
>>
>> *As a gymnast....*
>
> *That was how everyone identified me. I was a strong athlete and a good student but that is because I wouldn't have had it any other way. My coaches expected it, my mother expected it, and so it had to be. Some days I was so tired from going to school all day, getting picked up and eating my "early dinner," Than once I got to gym, the studio, the pool, I quickly changed into uniform. This left me 20 minutes to fix my hair and do as much homework as possible. It is 4:00 now, time to condition. It's 9:00 pm now and time to go home. But that means homework and my mind is racing on the drive home. My routine was horrible tonight, I should have been faster, and why is she better than me? Then I tell myself I will do better tomorrow, I MUST be better tomorrow. Home, shower; eat a little while I do my homework. It's 11:30pm, LIGHTS OUT! Sleep as much and as quickly as I can and make sure my alarm is set at 5:00am so I can finish my homework and start the day all over. But I'm an athlete, and that is what you do, that is what I must do...*

Males and Eating Disorders

Eating disorders are less common in men: approximately 10% of those suffering from eating disorders are males. Most likely this statistic is on the low end as there remains an old misconception that males cannot suffer from an eating disorder. There are many reasons that may further explain the low statistics of men suffering from eating disorders. Some of these include:

- Societal messages

- Lack of understanding from peers, siblings, and parents (quite often the primary male caretaker)

- Lack of male specific treatment groups and treatment

Societal messages confirm that a prejudice or ignorance is still alive and well. Some of the messages that numerous males I have worked with received, include: "there is something wrong with you" or "you are pathetic or weak" or "are you kidding, that is something a girls go through, not boys." Males are often labeled as weak, effeminate, or homosexual. In addition, there may be protective layers of secrecy because of the lack of treatment groups and treatment centers designed for males. Often times, males with eating disorders are reluctant or resistant to participating in support groups because the groups are mostly composed of females. On the other hand, females may also express apprehension to share in a group setting that includes a male. If a therapist is skilled and knowledgeable in these dynamics, such group therapy can be a powerful therapeutic experience for all participants.

While men may not strive for "thinness" as often as in women, they will often lose weight in attempt to appear lean and muscular as a result of dramatically decreasing their body fat. A man's obsession with weight and appearance may be achieved through excessive exercise and even steroid use. These behaviors are viewed as more acceptable, worthy of praise, and even "normal." In addition, if it turns into a preoccupation for physical perfection then it is likely to be considered risky, unhealthy, and potentially dangerous. Studies have also showed that certain athletic activities appear to put males at higher risk for developing an eating disorder. Sports which differentiate athletes by weight brackets, such as horse racing, wrestling, and boxing, are accompanied by an increased risk for developing an eating disorder such as anorexia or bulimia. The pressure to be competitive and to win at all costs, combined with non-athletic pressures in their lives creates a potential for the development of eating disorders.

We must continue to create an environment where males can feel safe and understood, and can be accepted without judgment so they no longer need to suffer in silence. Our society is gradually becoming more aware that eating disorders can occur in men too; however, there is still a long way to go.

Severity and Prevalence of Eating Disorders

In the United States, **as many as 10 million females and 1 million males** are fighting a life and death battle with an eating disorder such as anorexia or bulimia. **Millions more** are struggling with binge eating disorder. [16, 23, 42, 91] As a result of the secretiveness and shame associated with eating disorders, many cases are probably not reported. In addition, many individuals struggle with body dissatisfaction and sub-clinical disordered eating attitudes and behaviors. For example, 80% of American women are dissatisfied with their appearance.[94] The following statistic was gathered from a nationally representative face-to-face household survey (n=9282), conducted in 2001-2003, who were assessed using the WHO Composite International Diagnostic Interview:

- Lifetime prevalence estimates of DSM-IV anorexia nervosa, bulimia nervosa, and binge eating disorder are .9%, 1.5%, and 3.5% among women, and .3%, .5%, and 2.0% among men.[44]

In a 2003 review of the literature, Hoek and van Hoeken[43] found:

- Forty percent of newly identified cases of anorexia are in girls 15-19 years old.

- Significant increase in incidence of anorexia from 1935 to 1989, especially among young women aged 15-24.

- A rise in incidence of anorexia in young women aged 15-19 in each decade since 1930.

- The incidence of bulimia in 10-39 year old women TRIPLED between 1988 and 1993.

- Only one-third of people with anorexia receive mental health care.

- Only 6% of people with bulimia receive mental health care.

- The majority of people with severe eating disorders do not receive adequate care.

In their lifetime, an estimated 0.6% of the adult population in the U.S. will suffer from anorexia, 1% from bulimia, and 2.8% from a binge-eating disorder.[44] These statistics, however, do not show an even distribution throughout the population:

- Women are much more likely than males to develop an eating disorder. They are three times as likely to experience anorexia (0.9% of women versus 0.3% of men) during their life. They are also 75% more likely to have a binge eating disorder (3.5% of women versus 2.0% of men).[44]

- The mortality rate among people with anorexia has been estimated at 0.56% per year, or approximately 5.6% per decade, which is about 12 times higher than the annual death rate due to all causes of death among females aged 15-24 in the general population.[97]

Additional statistics:

- Over one-half of teenage girls and nearly one-third of teenage boys use unhealthy weight control behaviors such as skipping meals, fasting, smoking cigarettes, vomiting, and taking laxatives.[105]

- Men are less likely to seek treatment for eating disorders because of the perception that they are a "woman's disease."

- Girls who diet frequently are 12 times as likely to binge as girls who do not diet.[70]

—2—

EARLY WARNING SIGNS

What we see depends mainly on what we look for.

-*Sir John Lubbock*

Many people are unable to spot the early warning signs of an eating disorder because they do not know what to look for. To complicate things, any individual suffering from an eating disorder quickly becomes an expert at hiding it. Part of having an eating disorder is suffering in silence and keeping secrets. If confronted, they will typically try to explain and rationalize their disordered eating behaviors. However, if these behaviors continue, the signs and symptoms become increasingly obvious and difficult to deny. In order to intervene sooner rather than later, one must know the early danger signs that may be indicative of a potential eating disorder. In this chapter, we will categorize a variety of behaviors to better recognize and understand what may be indicative of the early warning signs of an eating disorder. These areas include relationship with food, preoccupation with body, weight, and appearance, unhealthy weight control behaviors, physical changes, shifts in mood and relationships, as well as other self-harming or destructive behaviors.

The whole phenomenon does not develop overnight, but may instead start with disordered eating that has the potential to develop into a clinical eating disorder. Disordered eating is a term used to describe irregular eating behaviors or patterns, which, generally do not warrant an actual eating disorder. It is important to point out that disordered eating can include symptoms of anorexia, bulimia, binge eating disorder, which makes this type of eating equally as dangerous. It is also imperative to note that anyone and everyone who may struggle with disordered eating is at increased risk for developing a clinically diagnosable eating disorder.

Relationship with food

Relationship with food is a powerful assessment tool which can provide a great deal of information to assess for disordered eating and actual clinical eating disorders. An individual's relationship with food may reveal signs of a potential eating problem. This can be seen if one becomes preoccupied with food, displays unusual eating behaviors, and engages in food rituals.

Preoccupation with Food

Preoccupation with food may begin to be displayed as an extreme or excessive concern with or an intensified interest in food. The individual may start by talking more about various aspects of food, displaying an increased interest in cooking, and/or spending more time examining nutritional levels, including calorie counting. The person may be continually trying new diet fads and distinguishing foods as "good" or "bad." Preoccupation with food may also include bingeing. *Bingeing* refers to eating large amounts of food in short periods of time. Some warning signs of bingeing are finding many wrappers, empty food packages, or hidden stashes of high caloric food.

31

Unusual Eating Behaviors and Food Rituals

Unusual eating behaviors and food rituals may be an early warning sign of disordered eating which may in turn lead to an eating disorder. Any obsessive or ritual-like behaviors at mealtimes, such as spreading food around the plate, chewing slowly or eating very rapidly, spitting already been chewed food, or cutting food into tiny pieces are cause for concern. Additional examples include increased use of condiments on food, refusal to eat too many food types at one meal, or beginning to limit food choices. Some of these food behaviors may happen only once in a while, and may not evolve into an eating disorder, but knowledge may be the reason that it stops right there.

Preoccupation with weight, body, and appearance

Preoccupation with weight, body and appearance means spending excessive amounts of time ruminating on weight, body, and appearance. Below is a list of various ways that this preoccupation may manifest:

- *Constantly looking at self in the mirror* can become incredibly intrusive and extremely exhausting when it becomes constant. There is obviously nothing unusual about looking in the mirror. However, if it begins to interfere with other areas of functioning, then it may be an early warning sign that an individual is becoming increasingly body-obsessed. For example, if looking at oneself in the mirror involves continually turning to view oneself from every angle and then doing it again but this time breathing in, then the cause for concern increases.

- *Discomfort surrounding body* can become an extreme source of depression and anxiety. Some examples of behaviors which may be indicative of discomfort surrounding one's body include constantly touching parts of your body that you are dissatisfied with, or moving clothing so it does not actually touch particular body parts. More specific examples of this is stretching the bottom of the shirt to make sure the stomach is not protruding, or wearing layers of clothing or clothing that is too large.

- *Body checking,* a continuous "need" to check one's body, can manifest in numerous ways. Some examples include measuring one's wrist size by putting the other hand around it, feeling one's collarbones, or touching one's waist to make sure of being able to feel each and every bone.

- *Weighing self regularly* can become dangerous if that scale is becoming an indicator of one's mood for the day, or if it is being used more and more frequently, then this may be a concern.

- *Only wanting to talk about body, weight and appearance of self and others* can result in an increasingly limited conversation. Of course, in our society, focus on all of these areas is everywhere, including the front of every gossip magazine, on the photos being passed around online, in the talk over lunch, and in general, throughout our most popular media. Such talk, if excessive and restrictive, and if it becomes the primary and eventual sole topic of discussion, it may be an early warning sign of a potential or actual disorder.

- *Comparing oneself to others* is of course common and appropriate to pay attention and notice those around us. It is in fact important to see oneself in relation to others. However, this becomes a definite cause of concern if the behavior is accompanied by or followed by negative thoughts and feelings about oneself.

Unhealthy weight control behaviors refers to the actual tactics that are used to ignore, minimize, and distract one from their hunger cues as well as the means to control weight. These include, but are not limited to:

- *Purging* refers to trying to rid the body of calories from recently eaten food, by vomiting, laxatives, diuretics, diet pills, and excessive exercise. In regards to vomiting, a sign is leaving the table halfway through the meal to use the bathroom and turning on running water to mask sounds of vomiting. Another cause of concern would be if one returns to the table after the bathroom visit with glazed eyes, throat clearing, and the avoidance of eye contact.

- *Exercising more frequently,* whether by running, walking, swimming or dancing, can be seen as more obvious weight control behaviors. However, if any of these activities begin to compromise other areas of one's life, it may be a cause for concern. The more subtle and covert behaviors that also deserve attention, and possibly intervention, include movement that lacks direction or purpose, as for example, pacing and walking around when it may be more appropriate to be sitting or focused on an activity. An even more specific example is seen when one has a task to work on or to complete such as homework or a project, and seems to be walking aimlessly. This is often done for the purpose of burning unwanted calories.

- *Excessive gum chewing*

- *Fluid loading/water loading* is drinking unusually large amounts of fluid which creates a sense of fullness. Many individuals have indicated that this behavior is utilized to decrease appetite and to induce the sensation of fullness. Caffeine in diet sodas or cigarette smoking is also known to work as an appetite suppressant.

- Finding the "perfect" excuse to avoid eating, such as sleeping, running urgent errands, or scheduling appointments during meal times.

- Complaints of physical ailments such as stomaches, headaches, or illness as a means to eat less and consequently control weight.

- Spending more time on the computer, finding a browsing history of pro-anorexia (proana) or pro-bulimia (promia) or some other web sites related to weight loss.

Physical Changes

Physical indicators of a potential eating disorder may range from extreme changes in physical appearance, to regular headaches, stomach pains, constipation, and regular flu-like symptoms. Some additional early physical warning signs are restlessness, insomnia, and lack of energy. These physical signs are seen in conjunction with changes in some or many of the eating behaviors noted previously. More obvious signs are significant weight loss, rapid weight gain, or a constant fluctuation in weight. The more severe the eating disorder, the more severe the physical complications become. It is critical to check with a doctor to discuss any worrisome physical changes. The primary care physician will help one to understand which physical effects may be age appropriate, and which may be of medical concern.

Shifts in Mood and Relationships

Shifts in mood and relationships: The criteria listed below are some of the symptoms of both mood and anxiety disorders, which were discussed in the prior chapter. All of these criteria are of concern even if they are not connected to body, weight, food, and appearance. However, if these are observable characteristics and are "surrounding body, weight, food, or appearance," this may be an early warning sign of disordered eating which can ultimately result in an eating disorder.

- Excessive worry or heightened anxiety "surrounding body, weight, food, or appearance."

- Beginning to isolate from family and friends "due to body, weight, food, or appearance."

- Increased sense of hopelessness or despair "surrounding body, weight, food, or appearance."

- Expression of shame or guilt "surrounding body, weight, food, or appearance."

- Diminished interest in previously enjoyed activities "due to body, weight, food, or appearance."

- Difficulties concentrating or indecisiveness "surrounding body, weight, food, or appearance."

- Extensive mood swings "surrounding body, weight, food, or appearance."

Self-harm or other self-destructive behaviors.

Self harm, also referred to as self injury, self-mutilation, or cutting, and other self-destructive behaviors are most often indicative of a deeper emotional issue that needs to be addressed. While the use of drugs or self-injurious behaviors such as cutting, hair pulling and skin picking does not directly correlate to an eating disorder; these behaviors are often seen in conjunction with eating disorders. This also includes an increase in impulsive and risk-taking behaviors ranging from the use of substances, excessively spending money, and sexual promiscuity. No matter how or when self-harming or other self-destructive behaviors are used, they must never be ignored and instead assessed by the appropriate treatment professionals.

All of these behaviors would be reason for concern and are most definitely a reason to open the lines of communication. In addition, much data suggests that eating disorders that begin during adolescence may have a more successful prognosis and likelihood for complete recovery than eating disorders that begin later in life. So, these warnings signs must be taken very seriously as early intervention may just save a life.

—3—

TYPES OF EATING DISORDERS

Anorexia Nervosa

I'm not starving myself...I'm perfecting my emptiness.

Anorexia Nervosa is a disorder characterized by self-starvation and excessive weight loss. The individual suffering from anorexia experiences an intense fear of weight gain. Any actual or perceived weight gain produces a horrifying fear of getting fat. The anorexic's perception of her body is distorted. The areas of the body representing maturity, femininity, and/ or sexuality are often the areas viewed as "Fat." The anorexic sufferer also experiences unrealistic expectations of self, extreme rigidity, and perfectionistic traits. These traits can most often be traced back to early childhood. Anorexia causes one to be in a constant state of depletion, feeling undeserving of love, protection, and nurturance. This depletion and lack of nourishment often results in feeling less than, unworthy and invisible.

We cannot survive without food, our body will deteriorate, and we will inevitably die without eating. Food is nourishment. So, when one denies self of food, one denies oneself of nourishment, and without food and nourishment, one denies oneself of life itself. In my work, I have seen anorexia nervosa being closely correlated to living in deprivation. Depriving self of food can correlate to not feeling deserving of "the nutrients life has to offer." This does not mean that someone struggling with anorexia literally wants to die, instead, metaphorically speaking, anorexia can be perceived as a slow suicide. Most individuals suffering from anorexia end up with a very restricted diet that is sometimes limited to only a few foods. There is also a subtype of anorexia nervosa who may regularly purge, even after the consumption of small amounts of food, through self-induced vomiting or the misuse of laxatives, diuretics, or enemas. The individuals suffering from anorexia engages in behaviors to disconnect from their bodily hunger cues, but actually obsesses about food all day long. These individuals deeply experience a strong yearning to control, deny, or disconnect from their desire to eat. Unhealthy and ritualistic behaviors are also very commonly used to try to control their weight or hunger. To the individuals suffering from anorexia, self-starvation and weight loss are viewed as a success, a sign of remarkable discipline and control over their life.

The following diagnostic criteria which define Anorexia Nervosa, are taken from The *Diagnostic and Statistical Manual of Mental Disorders, Fourth Edition, Text Revision (DSM IV-TR, 2000).*[3]

307.1 Anorexia Nervosa

A. Refusal to maintain body weight at or above a minimally normal weight for age and height, for example, weight loss leading to maintenance of body weight less than 85% of that expected; or failure to make expected weight gain during the period of growth, leading to body weight less than 85% of that expected.

B. Intense fear of gaining weight or becoming fat, even though underweight.

C. Disturbance in the way in which one's body weight or shape is experienced, undue influence of body weight or shape on self-evaluation, or denial of the seriousness of the current low body weight.

D. In postmenarcheal females, amenorrhea, i.e., the absence of at least 3 consecutive menstrual cycles. (A woman is considered to have amenorrhea if her periods occur only following hormone, e.g., estrogen administration).

Specify type:

Restricting Type: During the current episode of Anorexia Nervosa, the person has not regularly engaged in binge-eating or purging behavior (self-induced vomiting or the misuse of laxatives, diuretics, or enemas)

Binge Eating/Purging Type: During the current episode of Anorexia Nervosa, the person has regularly engaged in binge-eating or purging behavior (i.e., self-induced vomiting or the misuse of laxatives, diuretics, or enemas)

Case vignette of Anorexia Nervosa

Rachel, a 32 year old female, reported her first significant weight loss during her first year of college away from home. She had been in numerous treatment centers since that time and reports that recovery has been an ongoing struggle. Rachel had always been very athletic as a young girl. This included being a dancer as well as avid runner.

She had consistently been a good student and had placed very high expectations of herself from as long as she could remember. She has an incredible fear of being "fat" and will do whatever is needed and at all costs to prevent what she sees as the most horrific catastrophe possible, being "FAT." Rachel dresses in baggy clothes, wearing several layers, and describes her reasoning as being cold all of the time.

Rachel typically wakes up by 5:00 am, but on the weekend she allows herself to sleep until 5:30 am. She begins her day with a large cup of coffee from the same large cup she uses daily. She pours a splash of fat free creamer and uses 3 packets of an alternative sweetener along with one teaspoon of honey, but she insists that it must be one particular brand. Rachel then puts on her running shoes, rain or shine, and runs for 1.5 hours. Upon return, Rachel takes off her clothes and immediately steps on the scale. This will be her determining factor for the entire rest of her day, including her mood and her food intake. After she scrutinizes her body by touching her bones, measuring her wrist size, she proceeds to eat breakfast. This either consists of a 4 oz. bowl of oatmeal with several packets of an alternative sweetener along with a quarter cup of nonfat milk or a container of vanilla nonfat yogurt with 10 blueberries. Breakfast is followed by another weigh in and body check before she proceeds to shower and get ready for her day. Rachel sticks to a rigid regimen of no more than 550 calories a day. She only allows herself to eat specific foods at the same time every day. Her food choices have become increasingly limited over the many years she has struggled with anorexia.

Physical signs and symptoms of Anorexia

- Malnutrition
- Amenorrhea (loss of menses)
- Dizziness and headaches
- Bloating
- Abdominal pain
- Constipation
- Muscle weakness
- Excessive exercise
- Evidence of laxative, diet pills or diuretics to control weight
- Edema (water retention)
- Cold hands and feet
- Cold intolerance
- Hypersensitivity to noise and light
- Lethargy and/or excess energy
- Emaciation
- Pale complexion
- Noticeable thinning and loss of hair
- Dryness of skin/scalp
- Lanugo- increased facial and body hair
- Wearing baggy clothes to hide weight loss

Lanugo is the growth of fine, downy hair, similar to "peach fuzz", on the face and body. It is usually visible on the face first, but tends to appear in areas where there is typically very little hair growth, such as the face, chest and back areas. Lanugo grows on the human fetus while it is still in the womb, and is shed and replaced by a thicker hair the first few weeks of life. So, on the body of an individual suffering from anorexia, it is a primal attempt for the body to retain heat when the insulating effect of body fat is missing. This type of hair also takes fewer calories to produce than normal hair.

Case vignette of physical signs and symptoms of Anorexia:

Karen, a 23-year-old female, has been experiencing numerous physical signs and symptoms of anorexia nervosa. She has been noticing many changes to her body in addition to the expected weight loss. Her hair has begun thinning and falling out, especially whenever she brushes her hair. She has noticed that her skin is extremely dry and no matter how much of the lotion she applies, Karen's skin remains dry and unmosturized. She even went to get a manicure and noticed that even her nails were very brittle and breaking easily. In regards to her clothing, Karen is wearing many layers, no matter what the weather is as she complains of constantly being cold. In addition, she has great inconsistency with her sleep patterns, and is either easily fatigued, has little energy, or experiences the complete opposite.

Psychological signs and symptoms of Anorexia Nervosa

- Perfectionist traits, extreme difficulty with flexibility
- Depression
- Anxiety
- People with anorexia are not only afraid of food, but also afraid of themselves.

- Need to be in control
- Pursuit of thinness
- Isolated
- Diminished capacity to think
- Increased mood swings
- Rigidity in all thoughts, feelings, and experiences
- Inferiority, shame, and constant self-criticism
- A feeling of self worth determined by what is or is not eaten
- Noticeable discomfort around food

Case vignette of psychological signs and symptoms of Anorexia Nervosa

Karen noticed that she feels extreme anxiety when there is any change or disruption to her routine. Unfortunately for Karen, one never knows when life will just knock on the door with its physical illnesses and financial responsibilities. This anxiety may result in an increase of obsessive-compulsive behaviors and her need for control. This may ultimately result in feelings of inferiority and shame, which may lead to increased depressive symptoms and isolation.

Unhealthy Behaviors and Food Rituals

- Excessive gum chewing
- Tearing/cutting food into small pieces
- Covering food with extra condiment
- Collecting cookbooks or menus and cooking for other people

- Trying to shop for and feed other people
- Eating slowly, procrastinating, or playing with food
- Excessive talking, or no talking or eye contact at meals
- Eating foods in certain orders
- Excessive intake of fluids
- Weighing or measuring food
- Avoiding social eating
- Utilizing distracting behaviors such as working or shopping
- Excessive, rigid exercise routine despite weather, illness, or injury.
- Excuses for not eating meals (e.g. ate earlier, not feeling well)

Case vignettes of unhealthy weight control behaviors and food rituals

A. *I describe myself as a good friend, but sometimes I wish I didn't care so much. I will do whatever it takes to eat alone, but if I am in a position of going out with others and being in a restaurant, I will make any and all excuses to avoid eating. I will always order a drink so I feel somewhat a part of the company I am with, and I will be the one to do a great deal of the talking. I do this as a way to avoid focus being on restricting my food intake and to attempt to ensure the comfort level of those in my company.*

B. *I struggle with the tendency to assume what others are thinking and I know I display a great amount of rigidity surrounding my thoughts, feelings, and experiences. Even if someone I do or don't*

45

know looks at me, whom I may often construe
as staring at me, I already know what he or she is
thinking. I am convinced they look at me and say,
"Oh, look how fat she is" or "look how terrible
she looks." Either way, I know they are most
definitely thinking demeaning and judgmental
thoughts.

C. I thought being 100 lbs would make everything
better, but then I got there and it didn't get better,
so then thought that maybe if I made it to 95 lbs, I
will be happier then and only then, and it still did
not work. No matter how much weight I lost, even
down at 82 lbs, I still was not thin enough, happy
enough, in fact everything just kept getting worse.
But, I am still hoping maybe I will get something
better, whatever it is, at 75 lbs. When I started
this I couldn't think of anything but food, weight,
and appearance. I really believed I had become
consumed with all of that then, but now it is even
worse. I feel confused half the time; sometimes
I don't even make sense to myself. I can't really
think very clearly, I just want to be alone, I hate
myself and I am not good at anything. I can't even
do my eating disorder right, the voices never stop
in my head telling me how worthless I am, that I
don't deserve anything, especially food, and that
if I eat, I am just pathetic and fat.

Medical complications and consequences of Anorexia Nervosa

Self-starvation denies the body the essential nutrients it
needs to function normally resulting in serious medical
complications. Anorexia nervosa affects the entire body. This
includes the brain and nerves, the heart, the blood, muscles
and joints, kidneys, bodily fluids, intestines, hormones, and

the skin. Below is a list of specific medical complications and consequences of anorexia nervosa:

- Heart rhythm abnormalities
- The risk of heart failure rises as heart rate and blood pressure levels decrease.
- Osteopenia/Osteoporosis, which is the degenerative loss of bone density resulting from lack of calcium and other dietary deficiencies.
- Low potassium (most common cause of cardiac arrest)
- Severe dehydration that can result in kidney failure.
- Anemia (low red blood cell count)
- Severe electrolyte abnormalities
- Endocrine abnormalities-including mismanagement of diabetes
- Amenorrhea
- Cathartic colon (caused from laxative abuse)
- Infertility
- Death

Heart disease is the most common medical cause of death in people with severe anorexia nervosa. One can develop an irregular heartbeat known as **bradycardia.** Heart arrhythmias, abnormal rhythms or rates in the resting heart, may be increased with exercise, caffeine, dehydration, and electrolyte imbalances. The heart muscles begin to starve and actually lose size and shrink. This can result in decreased cardiac output and low blood pressure. The most serious result is death.

Bone loss is another medical complication of severe anorexia nervosa. Osteopenia, loss of bone minerals, may lead to osteoporosis, a more advanced loss of bone density. This can lead to brittle bones that can break easily as a result of a loss of calcium. Almost 90% of women diagnosed with anorexia experience osteopenia and 40% have osteoporosis. The bone loss is a direct result of hormonal changes, malnutrition and vitamin deficiencies.

The **Gastrointestinal** effects of anorexia, such as constipation and bloating, are a direct result of malnutrition and the underuse of the gastrointestinal tract. Constipation is a common medical complication resulting from anorexia. In fact, many cases of anorexia are actually diagnosed by a medical doctor when the individual seeks out treatment for severe constipation. Gastrointestinal mobility slows down and it takes longer for the gastric system to empty. Food sits in the stomach for longer periods of time, which results in increased bloating and stomachaches. It is a vicious cycle as the gastric problems such as constipation, bloating, and a sensation of early fullness all tend to suppress the urge to eat, thus speeding up the processes of weight loss and starvation.

Blood findings usually indicate anemia, low red blood cell count, and leukopenia, low white blood cell count. These changes may exhibit themselves through fatigue, weakness and dizziness.

There may also be severe negative effects on the **endocrine system,** including **thyroid dysfunction** and **amenorrhea.** In regards to thyroid function, patients with anorexia nervosa are often diagnosed with hypothyroid (low thyroid). Symptoms include hair loss, dry skin, hypothermia, and bradycardia. Amenorrhea, lack of menstruation, is correlated with weight loss, inadequate body fat content, or weight loss. Resumption of menses is often used as a marker of recovery from anorexia.

The majority of the medical complications of anorexia nervosa are reversible with nutritional rehabilitation and weight restoration. However, nutritional rehabilitation can be trying, both physically and psychologically. If an individual is severely malnourished, she may be at higher risk for *refeeding syndrome.* Refeeding syndrome consists of metabolic disturbances that occur as a result of nutritional rehabilitation to the severely malnourished anorexic.

Awareness of refeeding syndrome is of upmost importance to ensure physical safety.

During weight restoration and metabolic recovery, it is not uncommon for one to retain more fluid becoming swollen and bloated. The physical discomfort of fluid retention and weight gain can lead to laxative abuse making it a vulnerable time for relapse to occur. On a psychological level, one may feel like they have lost their free will, actually believing that "they are making me gain this weight." So, while the majority of medical complications are reversible with slow refeeding and careful monitoring of body weight, heart rate and rhythm, and serum electrolytes; it takes time for the psychological development to catch up to the actual physical appearance. The greatest likelihood for successful recovery during this difficult time depends upon a strong support system and an experienced and cohesive treatment team.

Prevalence of Anorexia Nervosa

According to the National Eating Disorder Association (www.NationalEatingDisorders.org).[101] The following are statistics regarding the prevalence of anorexia:

- Between 0.5-1% of women suffer from anorexia.

- Between 5-20% of individuals struggling with anorexia nervosa will die. The probabilities of death increase within that range depending on the length of the condition.[71]

P.F., Sullivan (1995)[97], published the following statistics:

- For females between 15 and 24 years of age who suffer from anorexia nervosa, the mortality rate associated with the illness is 12 times higher than the death rate of ALL other causes of death.[97]

- Anorexia nervosa has the highest premature fatality rate of any mental illness.[97]

Bulimia Nervosa

Bulimia Nervosa, often referred to as bulimia, is a serious eating disorder characterized by a destructive and recurring pattern of binging, eating large amounts of food in a short period of time, followed by inappropriate compensatory behaviors to prevent weight gain. Those who suffer from bulimia nervosa commonly live in a world of shame, secrecy, and self-disgust. Binges most often occur in private and are accompanied by a sense of lack of control. According to the *Diagnostic Statistical Manual of Mental Disorders, Fourth Edition, Text Revision (DSM IV-TR, 2000)*,[3] this sense of lack of control is defined by a feeling that one cannot stop eating or control what or how much one is eating. In addition, in the all-or-nothing thinking of bulimics, any slip-up is a total failure. So, since one has failed anyway, why not go ahead and engage in an all-out binge? However, if there is any enjoyment or even a sense of disconnect before or during the binge, it is quickly replaced by feelings of guilt, shame, disgust, and self-loathing. Once the binge episode ends, the purging behaviors begin. The *Diagnostic Statistical Manual of Mental Disorders*[3] describes these behaviors as self-induced vomiting, misuse of laxatives, diuretics, enemas, or other medications, fasting, and/or excessive exercise. Fasting may often take place on the day following a binge.

The period of time between a binge and a purge is connected with high anxiety, intense desperation, and extreme feelings of guilt and shame. Bulimics may purge in a desperate attempt to burn off the calories following a binge. This may be because they feel overwhelmed in coping with their emotions and are looking for a way to punish themselves. Yet because they have so much shame after a binge, purging becomes a relief. It may be shameful to be in the cycle of binging and purging, but in the moment, purging seems far less shameful than eating too much and actually digesting the food. The obsession with food before the binge even takes place, the actual binge-and-purge episode, followed by trying to deal with the aftermath of it, is all extremely time-consuming. There is little time left to be productive, and this behavior becomes insidious to the core. Those suffering from bulimia are with usually within the normal weight range and may even look relatively healthy. This factor contributes to why bulimia nervosa is more difficult to identify in primary care settings. Those struggling with bulimia may hide their symptoms pretty well, most of the time, but that does not mean that the symptoms are not there. It is of extreme importance that treatment providers be aware of the often-silent presentation of this disease. As the disease progresses, the signs become more apparent and bulimia takes over a person's life. It compromises a person's body, consumes time and money, limits relationships, and narrows emotions to those that support the disorder itself. Bulimia nervosa has a profound effect on the body, and can have severe, even life-threatening medical complications.

The following are the Diagnostic Criteria from the *Diagnostic Statistical Manual of Mental Disorders, Fourth Edition, Text Revision, (DSM IV-TR, 2000):*[3]

307.51 Bulimia Nervosa

A. Recurrent episodes of binge eating. An episode of binge eating is characterized by both of the following:

(1) Eating, in a discrete period of time (e.g., within any 2-hour period), an amount of food that is definitely larger than most people would eat during a similar period of time and under similar circumstances.

(2) A sense of lack of control over eating during the episode (e.g., a feeling that one cannot stop eating or control what or how much one is eating).

B. Recurrent inappropriate compensatory behavior in order to prevent weight gain, such as self-induced vomiting; misuse of laxatives, diuretics, enemas, or other medications; fasting; or excessive exercise.

C. The binge eating and inappropriate compensatory behavior both occur, on average, at least twice a week for 3 months.

D. Self-evaluation is unduly influenced by body shape and weight.

The disturbance does not occur exclusively during episodes of Anorexia Nervosa.

Specify type:

Purging Type: during the current episode of Bulimia Nervosa, the person has regularly engaged in self-induced vomiting or the misuse of laxatives, diuretics, or enemas.

Nonpurging Type: during the current episode of Bulimia Nervosa, the person has used other inappropriate compensatory behaviors, such as fasting or excessive exercise, but has not regularly engaged in self-induced vomiting or the misuse of laxatives, diuretics, or enemas.

Case vignette of Bulimia Nervosa

When Laura was 18, she went away to college. She made friends, went to her classes, and went to parties with her peers. Laura was living in the dorm with several other girls. She found herself continually comparing herself to all of them. Watching them undress, she eyed their "skinny and perfect bodies" and thought "why can't I be like that?" Laura listened to them talk about a new diet every week, and participated in every new trend. No matter how hard she tried, Laura "never" felt enough next to all of these other girls. Thoughts like these began to consume her. These were not new thoughts or feelings, but they had never been so intense. This being Laura's first time away from home, she thought that the freedom was going to be incredible. She did not anticipate the response she was experiencing, how lonely she would actually feel or the competitiveness that would consume her.

But one day, Laura came home from class early only to find candy wrappers, a pizza box, and an empty pint on ice cream sitting on her bed. Next, she heard someone gagging in the bathroom and Laura immediately knew what she was up too. Laura quickly left the room, as she wanted to avoid any confrontation with her roommate. The thoughts raced through her mind. "Now I know how she stays so thin. I can do that and I can eat more. I don't have to do these stupid diets anymore. Maybe I have finally found the cure. I can eat whatever I want, lose weight, and feel better. My life can get better and I will finally feel like I fit in and life can be good, really good." This was the beginning of the binge-purge cycle that would ultimately bring Laura to the lowest point she ever experienced in her lifetime.

In the beginning, it felt like Laura's dreams were coming true. Laura had a secret. She believed she had it all under control and had found the answer to happiness. She could eat whatever she wanted, and she did, and she could vomit it all away afterwards. Laura began to spend the majority of her money on food. Laura would consume her food so quickly and eat until she felt so full and so sick that all she wanted to do was go to sleep.

That was not an option until she vomited and there was nothing left to come up. Throwing up became easier and easier but increasingly difficult to hide. Desperation set in, and Laura would vomit into plastic bags and cups, at times not throwing them away for days at a time.

Yet, as quickly as she believed she had found the answer, everything fell apart because Laura found that every part of her life was affected. Laura became completely preoccupied with thoughts of food, weight, and appearance. Her bingeing and purging became her best friend and her worst enemy. Laura's friendships became distant and even more shallow, her grades began to drop, she became short tempered with her parents each time she spoke with them on the phone, and she began to have constant headaches and sore throats. To make matters worse, Laura was not even losing weight. "Wasn't this why I started this in the first place?" Things that were of value and importance to Laura suddenly did not seem to matter anymore. The shame and guilt lead Laura into feeling more despair and anxiety. All of these factors only fueled that cycle. Only one thing seemed to quiet her head, and so she thought, made her feel better, well at least for a moment, and that was bingeing and purging.

Signs and Symptoms of Binge Eating

It is of relevance to note that the bulimic's idea of a binge may not be, and most likely is not, the same as another's idea of a binge. A binge may be very subjective in nature. Although a binge is loosely defined as a large consumption of calories in a brief period of time, bulimics tend to define binges by the type of food consumed and their mood state during this time period, not necessarily by the actual caloric intake.[34,87] There is a belief that more food was eaten than should have been consumed along with a simultaneous sense of lack of control. Below is a more specific list of the signs and symptoms associated with bulimia nervosa:

- Lack of control over eating

- Secrecy surrounding eating (i.e. going out alone on unexpected food runs or going to the kitchen after everyone is asleep.)

- Alternating between eating unusually large amounts of food and fasting.

- Disappearance of food (i.e. hidden stashes of junk food, empty wrappers)

- Hoarding food

Signs and Symptoms of Purging

- Going to the bathroom or leaving for a period of time after eating.

- Disguising sounds so no one can hear the vomiting (i.e. running the faucet).

- Smell of vomit on breath or the smell of mouthwash or mints

- Using laxatives, diuretics, or enemas after eating. Also may be using diet pills.

- Excessive exercise, despite weather, illness, or injury, especially following eating.

- "Chipmunk cheeks" appears as swelling in one's face. This condition is caused when one's lymph nodes and salivary glands swell up from excessive bingeing and purging.

- Calluses on the back of the hands and knuckles from self-induced vomiting.

- Discoloration or staining of the teeth due to stomach acid.
- Chronic sore throat or hoarseness
- Red eyes or broken blood vessels in the eyes
- Frequent fluctuations in weight

Case vignettes of purging

A. *I have to get rid of my food after I binge as quickly as I can. I will do whatever I need to do to make sure it gets out of my body and I feel that relief. I take my fingers, my index and middle finger, and stick them in my throat. I gag and then I vomit and vomit until I can vomit no more. I need to feel empty and I don't stop until nothing else comes up. I think I feel relieved but I also feel exhausted, ashamed, and dizzy and my throat hurts.*

B. *I learned how to keep my secret. I regularly ran water in the sink to cover the sound of my vomiting. At times, I would take a shower and vomit into the drain. Sometimes, I would walk down the street and puke in bushes or get in my car and drive to the closest gas station that I knew had a private stall. It did not matter where, all that mattered is I must.*

C. *I restricted, then binged and purged, then restricted, and then binged and purged. This cycle went on for a couple of years. But then, I found laxatives. Laxatives by no means became a replacement to my other eating disorder behaviors, but instead an "enhancement" to my regimen. I quickly became dependent on laxatives, at times taking up to 40 a day. I had already isolated myself, but this magnified it to the point that I could barely leave my home but only to buy food and more laxatives. I could not be any place for too long because my stomach constantly rumbled, nonstop gas, continuous abdominal pains, and I never knew when I would need to get to the bathroom immediately.*

D. *I read in a magazine about people using laxatives as a way of purging themselves. I had tried vomiting but couldn't do it. I started taking laxatives because I was scared that because I was eating so much I would get fat really quickly. I thought that if I took laxatives all the food would go straight through me. So when I first went out and bought some laxatives, I downed ten after my binge. I knew deep down that they did not really do anything to counteract the binge, but they made me feel empty and cleansed inside. It has been 10 years since I tried my first laxative and now I am up to 25 a day. I don't care what comes out of me as long as it is something.*

Emotional Signs and Symptoms of Bulimia Nervosa

Bulimic patients are characterized as extroverted perfectionists who are self-critical, impulsive, and emotionally undercontrolled.[87] Bulimics also commonly binge in private, and some may plan binges and purges according to time of day and privacy issues. They may eat normally around friends and family but then binge at other times when alone. The more severe the bulimia becomes, the more one may modify daily schedules to be certain of time for bingeing and purging.

Below is a list of some of the emotional signs and symptoms associated with bulimia nervosa:

- Distorted negative body image
- Preoccupation with shape, weight, dieting, and control of food to the point that it interrupts daily functioning and is a primary concern.
- Feeling like one cannot stop or control one's eating behavior
- Withdrawal from usual friends and activities
- Creation of lifestyle schedules or rituals to make time for binge-and-purge sessions.
- Depression
- Anxiety

Case vignette of emotional signs and symptoms of Bulimia Nervosa

I stepped on the scale every time I walked by the bathroom. But, I didn't just step on it once; I removed my clothing piece-by-piece and stepped on the scale every time in between. Then, by the time I was pretty much naked I stared at body in the mirror. Holding in my stomach from the side. Then staring at my eyes in the mirror, I would tell myself that if I lost a pound, I had to vomit more and if I gained a pound, I had to vomit more and harder, and if my weight was the same, well then I wasn't trying hard enough and I better vomit more. You see, I could never win. I was doomed and this became my life.

Learn to speak with words, not numbers on a scale.

-Anonymous

Medical Complications and consequences of Bulimia Nervosa

According the *National Eating Disorder Association*[101], recurrent binge-and-purge cycles can damage the entire digestive system, and purge behaviors can lead to electrolyte and chemical imbalances in the body that affect the heart and other major organ functions. The health consequences of this include:

- **Electrolyte imbalances** that can lead to irregular heartbeats and possibly heart failure and death. Electrolyte imbalance is caused by dehydration and loss of potassium, sodium and chloride from the body as a result of purging behaviors. The electrolyte disturbance of most concern is hypokalaemia (low potassium) since it can lead to heartbeat irregularities. The loss of nutrients and fluids from purging can also lead to kidney stones and eventual kidney failure.

- **Esophageal complications** range from a possible tear known as Mallory-Weiss to a life-threatening rupture of the esophagus or stomach. Although esophageal rupture, also known as Boerhaave's syndrome, is rare, mortality is high, reaching approximately 20%. Classically, patients will have severe chest pain, painful swallowing, tachypnea (rapid breathing), and tachycardia (rapid heart rate), and a left-sided pleural effusion (buildup of fluid between the layers of tissue that line the lungs and chest cavity), which shows up on a chest x-ray.[60,67] The passageway can become so narrow that it is difficult for food to pass through or it can rupture, requiring immediate surgery. Boerhaave's syndrome is the most lethal perforation of the GI tract. The best prognosis is with early diagnosis and definite surgical repair within 12 hours of rupture. Patients who undergo surgical repair within 24 hours of injury have a 70-75% chance of survival. This falls to 35-

50% if surgery is delayed longer than 24 hours and to approximately 10% if delayed longer than 48 hours.[60] Left untreated the mortality rate is close to 100%.[60] As with anything, the longer one has been engaging in these behaviors, the greater long-term risks where these medical complications can be potentially irreversible.

- Patients with bulimia nervosa often complain of heartburn and acid-reflux symptoms. Vomiting can also cause the stomach lining to become inflamed. Sometimes an individual even breathes in the vomit, which can damage the lungs. Another potential result from stomach acid is cold sores on and in the mouth. Stomach acid actually damages the soft tissue in and around one's mouth, which yes, leads to cold sores. This medical complication is very concerning, especially when it happens to an individual who is already faced with low self esteem, self-loathing, guilt and shame. as well as placing such a high value on appearance both to self and others.

- **Swelling of the salivary glands,** which are the glands surrounding the mouth that produce saliva, is a common medical complication. Often it is the parotid gland (the gland commonly affected in the mumps) that swells most, resulting in the face having a somewhat rounded, chubby appearance.[22] This condition is frequently referred to as chipmunk cheeks and does not a permanent effect. This condition should gradually decrease once the sufferer seizes the bulimic behaviors.

- **Anemia** is a condition caused by a low red blood cell count. A low amount of healthy red blood cells can mean one's body is not receiving enough oxygen. This results in symptoms such as fatigue, weakness, shortness of breath, feeling cold, increased infections, and heart palpitations.

- The most common **gastrointestinal symptoms** are bloating, flatulence, constipation, and chronic irregular bowel movements. Chronic irregular bowel movements and constipation as a result of laxative abuse.

- The most common **dental complications** include dental erosions, dental caries, and periodontal disease. The severity and rate of enamel loss may be related to numerous factors, such as duration of bulimia, frequency of purging, types of food consumed, quality of tooth structure, and oral hygiene.[60,102] Tooth decay and staining may also occur from stomach acids released during frequent vomiting.

- Irregular or absent period

- Oral complications of bulimia are primarily related to the chronic regurgitation of acidic gastric contents.[60] **Gum disease** (gingivitis) is also a direct result of chronic irritation from the acidic gastric contents and occurs as pain and inflamed red gums. Gum disease may not be one of the most serious medical complications, however, the emotional and financial stress that occurs as a result, makes it a very serious medical complication.

- Abrasions, calluses on the dorsum of the hand and knuckles, and scarring are the most characteristic **dermatologic** sign of self-induced vomiting done by inserting their fingers into their throat.[96]

- Laxative abuse can lead to lasting disruptions of normal bowel functioning and also produces a variety of fluid and electrolyte imbalances.[67] Laxative abuse can also damage the lining of the colon which may result in bloody stools or ulcers.

- Diuretic abuse can produce **fluid and electrolyte disturbance.**

- **Subconjunctival Hemmorage** is a medical term which refers to the rupture of blood vessels in the eyes which can result from extensive vomiting. I have seen clients in session actually start bleeding from the eye. The good news is that it does heal once the purging ceases, even though the psychological scars may be long lasting.

- Use of ipecac to induce vomiting can lead to extreme muscle weakness, including heart muscle weakness.

Prevalence and Facts of Bulimia Nervosa

- Bulimia nervosa affects 1-2% of adolescent and young adult women.

- Approximately 80% of bulimia nervosa patients are female.[32]

- People struggling with bulimia nervosa usually appear to be of average body weight.

- In bulimia nervosa, while vulnerability to obesity may put people at increased risk of developing the disorder, true obesity is rarely a problem. Rather, the key problem is the fear of obesity.[22]

- Many people struggling with bulimia nervosa recognize that their behaviors are unusual and perhaps dangerous to their health.

- Bulimia nervosa is frequently associated with symptoms of depression and changes in social adjustment.

- About one-fourth to one-third of bulimia nervosa patients have had a previous history of anorexia nervosa.[38]

- In addition to the full-blown disorder, symptoms of bulimia, such as occasional episodes of binge eating and purging occur in up to 40 percent of college women.[47,100]

Binge Eating Disorder

No matter what we weigh, those of us who are compulsive eaters have anorexia of the soul.

-Geneen Roth

Listed in the *Diagnostic Statistical Manual of Mental Disorders, Fourth Edition, Text Revision (DSM IV-TR, 2000)*[3] appendix as a diagnosis for further study, Binge Eating Disorder is defined as uncontrolled binge eating without emesis or laxative abuse. It is often, but not always, associated with obesity. Almost everyone overeats on occasion, and some of us may feel "too" full, and that we have eaten more than we should have. The individual suffering from Binge Eating Disorder, also referred to as BED, periodically goes on large binges, consuming an unusually large quantity of food in a short period of time (less than 2 hours), eating uncontrollably until they are uncomfortably full. Unlike bulimics, they do not purge or use compensatory measures following a binge episode.

Binge eating episodes are associated with three (or more) of the following:

(1) Eating much more rapidly than normal.

(2) Eating until feeling uncomfortably full.

(3) Eating large amounts of food when not feeling physically hungry.

(4) Eating alone because of being embarrassed by how much one is eating.

(5) Feeling disgusted with oneself, depressed, or very guilty after overeating.

People who suffer from binge eating disorder may vow again and again to stop, but they feel such a compulsion that they cannot resist their urges and continue bingeing. Some triggers for binge eating disorders include depression, anxiety, and trouble with interpersonal relationships, boredom, prolonged dieting, and body-image dissatisfaction. Many binge eaters (also known as compulsive overeaters) speak of using the coping skill of bingeing or "emotional eating" as ways to sedate, distract, or numb from them all that is going on around them. Many stuff food into their mouths almost mechanically, barely chewing it.[22] The binge may temporarily relieve the stress of these unwanted feelings, but unfortunately the binge is followed by intense feelings of shame, guilt, disgust, and further depression. One may even develop psychological and physical problems related to binge eating disorder. These problems contribute to creating even more misery and further reducing the quality of life. The sufferer may avoid work, school, or socializing with peers, due to the shame associated with the binge-eating problem, actual physical discomfort following a binge, or changes in their body shape and weight.

There are varying degrees of obesity resulting from binge eating disorder. While there is not a conscious choice to become obese, obesity may end up serving many functions. Obesity may serve as a way to create a larger body for protection and assist as a means to avoid physical intimacy. The more severe the obesity, the greater the risk of obesity-related health problems such as diabetes and sleep apnea.

Case vignette of Binge Eating Disorder

The minute I start thinking about food, I know I am in trouble. I try to stop the thoughts, but I can't. My thoughts move to specific foods, the ones I don't allow myself to eat when I am dieting. The urge gets stronger and stronger until I find myself in the kitchen eating, quickly. First, it tastes good, it feels good, and I think of nothing else. But soon, the comfort I felt moves to feeling sick, repulsed, guilty, and ashamed. Somehow, I make it to my bed and quickly fall asleep. Then comes the morning after...

Our greatest weakness lies in giving up. The most certain way to succeed is always to try one more time.

-Thomas Edison

Signs of Binge Eating Disorder

These signs include but are not limited to

- A pattern of eating in response to emotional stress, such as family conflict, peer rejection, or not meeting the expectations of self or others.

- Shame and disgust following a binge. Wanting to hide and be alone

- Finding food containers or wrappers hidden in various places.

- An increasingly irregular eating pattern, such as skipping meals, eating lots of junk food, and eating at unusual times.

Medical Complications and Psychological Consequences

- Depression, anxiety, panic attacks

- Social phobia

- Obesity

- High blood pressure

- Type 2 diabetes

- High cholesterol

- Gall bladder disease

- Heart disease

- Osteoarthritis

- Joint pain

- Gastro intestinal problems

- Sleep apnea

Prevalence and Facts of Binge Eating Disorder

- The only reliable way to find out whether binge eating causes obesity or vice versa is to track how people change over time to discover which comes first.[22]

- The prevalence of BED is estimated to be approximately 1-5% of the general population.

- Binge eating disorder affects women slightly more often than men—estimates indicate that about 60% of people struggling with binge eating disorder are female, 40% male.[93]

- People who struggle with binge eating disorder can be of normal or heavier than average weight.

- Binge eating disorder is associated with current severe obesity (body-mass index<_40).[44]

- BED is often associated with symptoms of depression

- People struggling with binge eating disorder often express distress, shame, and guilt over their eating behaviors.

Eating Disorder Not Otherwise Specified (EDNOS)

There is another diagnosis known as Eating Disorder Not Otherwise Specified (EDNOS), which involves disordered eating patterns. The EDNOS category is for disorders of eating that do not meet the criteria for any specific eating disorder. So, this diagnosis in the *Diagnostic Statistical Manual* is utilized when the sufferer does not "perfectly" fit the diagnoses of Anorexia Nervosa or Bulimia Nervosa. The following are the criteria according to the *Diagnostic Statistical Manual of Mental Disorders, Fourth Edition, Text Revision (DSM IV-TR 2000):*[3]

307.50 Eating Disorder Not Otherwise Specified

(1) For females, all of the criteria for Anorexia Nervosa are met except that the individual has regular menses.

(2) All of the criteria for Anorexia Nervosa are met except that, despite significant weight loss, the individual's current weight is in the normal range

(3) All of the criteria for Bulimia Nervosa are met except that the binge eating and inappropriate

compensatory mechanisms occur at a frequency of less than twice a week or for duration of less than 3 months.

(4) The regular use of inappropriate compensatory behavior by an individual of normal body weight after eating small amounts of food (e.g., self-induced vomiting after consuming two cookies).

(5) Repeatedly chewing and spitting out, but not swallowing, large amounts of food.

(6) Binge-eating disorder: recurrent episodes of binge eating in the absence of the regular inappropriate compensatory behavior characteristic of Bulimia Nervosa.

Of course, it is a good thing that the sufferer does not fit into the specific categories of eating disorder described above, but, on the other hand, it can also be very detrimental. I have seen this diagnosis send a dangerous message too the public far to many times, and it goes something like this...

"Oh I am not sick enough to get treatment."

"I can't even do my eating disorder good enough."

"I am not a bulimic, I am not anorexic, and so what am I?"

This diagnosis can also give sufferers a rationale for working harder at being exceptional at their eating disorder, especially if the eating disorder has become their identity. It has become far more widely accepted that an individual is suffering from an eating disorder well before they reach emaciation, stop having their period, or are bingeing and purging numerous times a day. Is their disorder sub-clinical? YES. Is it still serious enough to potentially cause death? YES! So, what happens when you are not "sick" enough to get help? It is already difficult enough to ask for help. However, the diagnosis is only a label, and one does not need to have a "neat" clinical diagnosis to get help. Let us examine a typical example of such a case to gain a deeper understanding:

Case vignette of Eating Disorder Not otherwise Specified (EDNOS)

I restricted, I binged, and I exercised compulsively, I was scared to death of food, and I had a horrible body image. I was obsessed with my weight and the amount of calories I put into my body, feeling like this defined who I was. I even used diet pills and laxatives. When I looked in the mirror I thought I was huge, but I was not "medically" considered underweight or overweight. So, even though I restricted, was terrified of food, had many bizarre food rituals, I never "qualified" as anorexic.

As stated earlier, in order to diagnose EDNOS, the clinician must first rule out the diagnoses of anorexia nervosa and bulimia nervosa. Individuals diagnosed with EDNOS may exhibit all of the signs of anorexia, but still have a regular menstrual cycle or may lose weight, but still continue in the normal weight range. Others may have all the symptoms of bulimia, but will not binge or purge as often as is required to be categorized as having bulimia. Many people diagnosed with EDNOS also exhibit other symptoms associated with anorexia, bulimia, or binge-eating such as:

• Purging, or compensating for normal eating by inducing vomiting, using laxatives or over-exercising, but not doing it enough to be diagnosed with one of the clinical eating disorders

- Binge eating regularly and compensating for it through the use of laxatives or by vomiting

- Remaining within their normal weight range despite disordered eating

- Eliminating entire food groups from their diet (and that includes carbohydrates!)

- Being preoccupied with exercising, but eating fairly regularly

- Believing that everyone is as focused on one's weight as one is

- Chronic dieting, always on or off or going on a diet

- Obsessing with eating only organic, natural, or raw foods (orthorexia)

—— 4 ——

THE MULTI-DISCIPLINARY TREATMENT APPROACH

Unity for Successful Treatment

*Nobody can do everything, but
everyone can do something.*

-Anonymous

No one type of treatment can operate independently for successful recovery from an eating disorder. There are far too many components of treatment that require the expertise of many professionals. Creating a treatment team the patient feels comfortable and safe with is of prime importance. The team must be willing to communicate with each other and to create an-ongoing treatment plan that is in the best interest of the client. If the patient is being treated on an outpatient basis, each member of the team most likely works independently in separate treatment locations. This is acceptable for so long as the treatment-providers are open to working with others. If a treatment provider has any apprehension about this approach or does not have experience in the treatment of eating disorders, then one may want to re-evaluate this provider's participation.

Professionals from several disciplines who are experienced in the treatment of eating disorders may collaborate in a patient's care. Each treatment provider brings unique expertise to the team. If the patient is an adolescent, it is especially important that treatment providers be knowledgeable about normal adolescent physical and psychological growth and development. This interdisciplinary team may include, but is not limited to, a primary care physician, a registered dietitian, a psychiatrist, mental health professionals, and other professionals as needed (i.e., cardiologist, gastroenterologist, dentist, gynecologist).

Primary Care Physician

The primary care physician will monitor the patient's physical well being. A physician is able to rule out any medical illnesses, and to determine that the individual is not in any immediate medical danger. In addition, the physician can perform an initial assessment and continue to treat any potential medical complications.

A medical assessment should include a physical examination by a physician to assess all organ systems including dermatologic, gastrointestinal and cardiovascular, as well as endocrine function.[47,59] Laboratory tests should also be conducted and should routinely include serum electrolytes, creatinine, blood urea nitrogen, and a complete blood count. Radiographic or endoscopic assessment procedures may be needed for those with gastrointestinal bleeding along with additional tests for those with significant abdominal symptoms. Serum calcium and phosphate should also be conducted for individuals with chronic amenorrhea and emaciation.[59] Bone density studies may also be needed. The physician must establish a baseline for future comparisons.

In addition, since an initial step in treatment is to assess a patient's motivation to change, and since there is often apprehension about letting go of the eating disorder, the physician may be able to increase the patient's motivation as the patient gains more insight into the medical complications of eating disorders.

Registered Dietitian or Nutritionist

The role of the registered dietitian or nutritionist is a difficult one, since these are the ones dealing directly with food. It is the position of the American Dietetic Association[2] that nutrition intervention, including nutritional counseling by a registered dietitian, is an essential component of the team treatment of patients with anorexia nervosa, bulimia nervosa, and other eating disorders during assessment and treatment across the continuum of care. The dietitian helps each individual develop an individualized meal plan, discusses lab test results with the physician, and assists in finding ways nutrition can be utilized for more effective treatment. The dietitian also provides education on a healthy diet and on identifying appropriate weight goals. In addition, these professionals have the capacity to evaluate diets and to make changes based on an individual's medical condition, physical activity, food preferences, and religious beliefs. Additionally, the dietitian will evaluate whether food beliefs and behaviors fall into what might be considered the normal range.[2]

A nutritional assessment will have different components depending on the stage of illness and treatment setting. The assessment should include a weight history, including the patient's current, highest, and lowest body mass index, and nutrient deficiencies, typical current daily food intake, methods of weight control, and physical activity. In addition, a nutritional assessment should include an evaluation of the patient's attitudes and perceptions about their body, including the size and shape of it overall, as well as specific body parts.[47,59]

Nutritionists and registered dietitians have a powerful role to play in that they are in a position to nurture the patient into a new way of developing a trusting relationship with food and body. Developing a trusting relationship with the patient is critical for successful treatment. This often takes time, as there are many challenges that this relationship will face. The needs of early recovery are not the same as those needed later in recovery. As the patient goes through changes with their bodies', meal plans may need to be adjusted.

Psychiatrist

The psychiatrist is certainly one of the most important members of the treatment team. Psychiatrists are medical doctors who are trained to perform various types of psychotherapy and prescribe psychotropic (mind altering) medication. The psychiatrist will assess if medication is needed for underlying mood or anxiety disorders, and to provide overall input for the most comprehensive individualized treatment possible. Psychiatrists will have an understanding of the biological aspects of eating disorders and related medical and psychological pathologies. Due to the high level of psychiatric conditions that go along with eating disorders, mood stabilization is a critical step to effective recovery.

Psychiatric medical management of eating disorders has shown to be very effective, but it has by no means proven to be a cure. The psychiatrist will usually not prescribe medication until the following treatments have commenced:

(1) Nutritional rehabilitation

(2) Psychoeducation and initiation of psychotherapy

(3) Any co-occurring disorders that may respond to medication are clearly identified, particularly when they existed prior to the onset of the eating disorder.

Therapist

It is critical that the treating psychotherapist, whether a psychologist or therapist, has a specialization or a great deal of experience in the treatment of eating disorders. For successful psychotherapy to take place, a safe, trusting, and nurturing therapeutic relationship must be established. In addition, the patient must be medically stable to be able to participate meaningfully in any type of psychological treatment.

Once the treating clinician has identified important issues that need attention, a treatment plan should be developed. To help establish and nurture the therapeutic relationship, the therapist should involve the client in establishing treatment goals. It is important to note that the therapist is working with the patient, not for the patient. Then, to ensure the likelihood of successful recovery from an eating disorder, the therapist and patient continue their work together to explore and resolve the psychological issues that give rise to the eating disorder.

Throughout the therapeutic process, trust will be an ongoing thread that holds the relationship between the therapist and the client together and allows the sufferer to heal and let go of the eating disorder. The therapist must listen to their patients, hear them, respect them, acknowledge them, nurture them, and teach them, so that they can learn to listen and trust themselves. The therapist must embrace, nurture, and teach their patients to break. through the unrelenting self-hatred and self-loathing, so they can learn how to self-soothe and gain self-respect. It is critical to work with the eating disorder sufferer to unveil their voice, which that individual only knows how to speak through eating disorder behaviors. It is the therapist's job to create, nurture and sustain a relationship in which the sufferer can constantly "refine the truths" she tells herself and others.[81] Therapy is a process of going deeper and deeper into the layers of oneself in order to discover how one lost their identity to the rules and commands of their eating disorder. It is a place and a relationship where the sufferer can tear down the wall that once provided protection from pain, rejection and invalidation, a place where her true authenticity is "enough." The therapeutic space becomes a sanctuary, a resting place where a kind of slow learning occurs.[95]

5

TYPES OF THERAPY

Your ranges of available choices--right now--are limitless

-Frederick Frieseke

Several different treatment modalities are utilized throughout the therapeutic process and they are tailored to the patient's needs. For instance, the patient may initially need to focus on establishing tools to tolerate the discomfort experienced in letting go of an eating disorder, prior to engaging in more introspective work. Some of these treatment modalities include psychoeducation, cognitive-behavioral therapy, dialectical-behavioral therapy, self-psychology, and motivational enhancement therapy.

Psychoeducation

Psychoeducation is a form of therapy that is strongly education based and is aimed at teaching and discussing with individuals the basic facts about all aspects of the eating disorder.

Cognitive Behavioral Therapy (CBT)

Cognitive Behavioral Therapy, CBT, is action-oriented and collaborative with the therapist and the patient. CBT assumes that maladaptive, faulty, or irrational beliefs and thinking patterns cause one to engage in maladaptive and self-destructive behaviors. The belief is that if one identifies, challenges, and replaces these maladaptive thoughts with rational thoughts, this will lead to reasonable emotions followed by constructive behaviors. This approach is quite fitting to the treatment of eating disorders because the cognitive components address the maladaptive thinking, also known as cognitive distortions, which goes along with eating disorders.[57,89] Some of these cognitive components include the extreme preoccupation about shape and weight, perfectionism, low self-esteem, all-or-nothing thinking, personalization, and overgeneralization. The behavior components of CBT identify and work to change the disturbed and destructive eating habits. Some examples include restricting, binging, purging, compensatory behaviors, excessive exercise, as well as isolation, procrastination, and avoidance.

Therapists utilizing CBT help patients learn to identify correctly their cognitive distortions, and then challenge the negative thinking, and ultimately disprove it. By challenging and replacing the negative thinking time and again, it will slowly diminish and be replaced by more rational, balanced thinking. The belief is that anything that is learned can be unlearned and relearned a new way. Listed below are some specific cognitive distortions along with an example that will explain further:

1. **Personalization**-When one sees oneself as the cause of some problem even if there is no indication or truth to confirm this belief. Personalization leads to feelings of guilt, shame, and inadequacy, and thoughts such as:

- *I am a disappointment to myself and to my mother especially when I make a mistake.*

- *It's my fault that my parents are fighting, I cause so many problems.*

2. **All-or-nothing thinking** - When one sees things in black and white categories. If one's performance falls short of perfect, one sees oneself as a total failure. This cognitive distortion is extremely prevalent when one has high, often unrealistic expectations of self, leading to thoughts such as:

   - *No matter what I do, it is never enough.*

   - *I have to weigh 90 lbs. to be enough*

   - *I can't ever get it right; no matter what, I am a complete failure.*

3. **Always being right** - Being wrong is unthinkable and one will do or say whatever is necessary to prove that one's opinions and actions are correct. This is a very close-minded attitude that does not allow space for others to have an opinion. This makes others frustrated and the end result is usually damaged and broken relationships.

4. **Should statements** - One tries to motivate oneself with should not statements, as if one had to be whipped and punished before one could accomplish anything. "Musts" and "ought's" also fall into this faulty-thinking category. The emotional consequence is shame and guilt.

   - *I should work today; no I really must work today even though I feel miserable. I am not sick enough to miss work.*

   - *I am kind of hungry but it will pass eventually so I should just wait.*

5. **Disqualifying the positive & Minimization** - One rejects positive experiences and successes by insisting that they do not count for some reason or other.

   - *I know I didn't purge today but it's no big deal because I have gone a day without purging before and then I end up screwing up the next day anyway.*

6. **Mind reading** - One is able to determine what another individual is thinking and how that individual is feeling, without the individual saying anything. For example, a person may conclude that someone is reacting negatively toward them and does not actually bother to find out if they are correct. One may predict a negative outcome and assume things will go negatively. Other examples under this category include jumping to conclusions and "fortune telling."

   - *I know they are all talking about me and saying how disgusting I look in my outfit.*
   - *I am going to mess up on this interview and not get this job.*
   - *I asserted myself but I am sure they probably thought I was stupid for what I said anyway.*
   - *I know she is talking about me and saying how fat I am.*

7. **Blaming** - Blame is the opposite of personalization, where one does not take any responsibility and claims "it is everyone else's fault." This tends to keep individuals in a "victim" role or can even make them believe they are better than everyone else.

   - *It's my mother's fault that I have this eating disorder*
   - *It's because he broke up with me that I have been cutting.*

8. **Overgeneralization** - Coming to a general conclusion based on a single incident or piece of evidence.

   - *See, she didn't even call me back, I will never have any friends and I will always be alone.*

   - *If I eat more calories that I think I should have, that means I am a failure and if I can't even do my anorexia perfect, than I will be miserable forever.*

   - *If I gain one pound, I will be completely and utterly fat.*

9. **Mental Filter** - This is characterized by focusing solely on a single negative detail while ignoring positive ones.

   - *My dietitian told me that I am doing so much better following my meal plan, but that I am not practicing enough flexibility with my food choices. All I can focus on is that I am not doing it good enough, not that I am doing so much better.*

10. **Emotional reasoning** - Here one believes that what one feels must be true.

   - *I believe it, I feel it, and therefore it must be true.*

   - *I feel pathetic and worthless; therefore I am pathetic and worthless.*

11. **Catastrophizing** - No matter what, one expects the worst outcome.

   - *I did horrible at gymnastics today; I am never going to get that skill; I am really pathetic; what's the point, maybe I should just quit gymnastics because I am never going to make it to the next level and probably never going to make it to a college scholarship.*

In summary, these cognitive distortions lead to feelings of depression and anxiety; they result in all types of destructive behaviors from eating disorder behaviors to isolation and avoidance. These distortions inevitably alienate friends and family, and they leave one completely alone. When a sufferer identifies an automatic negative thought (i.e., a cognitive distortion), the sufferer must challenge the thought even if this person does not believe it at the times. It takes a great deal of practice. Below is an example:

One has made plans to go out to eat with a friend. As the day progresses, one notices the onset of anxiety. One starts to connect to negative thoughts that are causing this anxiety.

- *Maybe I should cancel; it's not really like she will care anyway. (should, catastrophizing, fortune telling)*

- *I am so boring anyway and just bring everyone down. (personalization, all or nothing thinking, jumping to conclusions)*

- *Actually, she cancelled on me before so, I can actually cancel one time too. (blaming, mental filter, overgeneralization)*

- *I should have never made this plans because I always end up flakinganyway- I am such a flake and a bad friend. (shoulds. emotional reasoning, all or nothing thinking)*

So I begin to replace these thoughts as seen below:

- *My friend does care; the last time I cancelled she told me how sad she was and how much she misses me.*

- *I am actually a lot of fun and when I am present and engaged, I can even make others laugh.*

- *I would be lying if I cancel and being honest makes me feel good and is an integral part of my recovery.*

- I am a good friend and I made these plans because I deserve to have fun.

- Eating with others is actually enjoyable and every time I do it, it gets easier and easier.

When I think these thoughts, I actually feel calmer and even excited for my plans. So flaking is no longer an option. My friend knows that I am in recovery and has stayed by my side through it all. I am going to call my friend right now to let her know that I am looking forward to going out.

Dialectical Behavioral Therapy (DBT)

Dialectical Behavioral Therapy is also known as DBT. In this section, I will be providing a very broad overview of DBT. I encourage anyone who is interested in learning more to refer to the references section under Marsha Linehan.[57,58] Dialectical Behavioral Therapy, DBT, combines cognitive behavioral therapy while incorporating eastern mindfulness practices and placing high emphasis on validation and acceptance. Although acceptance of clients as they are is crucial to any good therapy, DBT goes a step further than standard cognitive-behavioral therapy in emphasizing the necessity of teaching individuals to fully accept themselves and their world as they are in the moment.[58] It is important to note that in the terminology of DBT, almost any desired behavior can be thought of as a skill. The central theme of DBT as a whole is to replace ineffective, maladaptive, or non-skilled behavior with skillful responses. DBT includes psychosocial skills training to help the individual acquire the needed skills through a progression of the following four modules:

1. **Mindfulness** has to do with the quality of awareness that we bring to what we are doing and experiencing to be in the here and now. DBT skills training module aims

to teach a core set of "mindfulness" skills, that is, skills having to do with the ability to consciously experience and observe oneself and surrounding events.

2. **Distress tolerance** behaviors targeted in DBT skills training are concerned with tolerating and surviving crises and overwhelming emotions with acceptance of life in the moment. There are simply times when thoughts, emotions, and situations are just too overwhelming, unsafe, or intolerable, to deal with. Since one is placed in situations that cannot be changed, and, for whatever reason, one does not feel or believe they have healthy tools to tolerate the discomfort and distress they are facing. The premise is not to become avoidant, or to suppress emotional pain, but instead get through a bad situation without making it worse. Four sets of crisis survival strategies are taught:

   • Distracting (through activities, contributing, comparisons, generating opposite emotions, pushing away from a situation, distracting with other thoughts, and creating sensations to interfere with the physiological component of the current negative emotion)

   • Self-soothing (by using each of the five senses)

   • Improving the moment (through imagery, meaning, prayer, relaxation, one thing in the moment, vacation, and encouragement)

   • Thinking of pros and cons (for both tolerating and not tolerating the discomfort).[58]

In addition, these skills are imperative to have in place when one is in the therapeutic process, being faced with continuous triggers when one has still not integrated new and healthy.

Getting through the crises without making it worse may be just the answer in that moment. The acceptance piece to distress tolerance does not mean one is "ok" with whatever one is faced with. It is instead about coming to terms with and accepting the premise that suffering and pain are indeed inevitable and a part of life. Trying to run from this truth only creates more pain and suffering. Learning to tolerate and accept distress skillfully by accepting actually leads to decreased pain and suffering, short and long term, and inevitably helps to "grant me the serenity to accept the things I cannot change, the courage to change the things I can, and the wisdom to know the difference.[1] (Serenity prayer)

3. **Emotional Regulation** deals with understanding the nature of emotions, learning how to identify and label emotions in everyday life, identifying the functions of emotions and their relationship to difficulties in changing emotions, reducing vulnerability to negative emotions, how to increase positive emotional events, and how to decrease emotional suffering through mindfulness to the current emotion and taking opposite action.[58] To better understand why this concept is so critical for the eating disorder sufferer, refer back to Chapter 2, psychological and emotional factors.

4. **Interpersonal Effectiveness** is another DBT skills training module that was developed in response to working with "borderline" individuals whose relationships are chaotic, intense, and marked with difficulties. I am sure we can all relate to some of these factors, but do remember that chaos and intensity lies on a continuum, and we can all benefit from some interpersonal effectiveness skills training.

Overall, each one of these skills has some overlap, each with the other, especially the mindfulness with all of the other skills. Either way, all of the skills come together in a synergistic way. These skills are taught and implemented in both individual and group therapy, with an extremely strong emphasis placed on the therapeutic relationship.

Family Therapy

The relationships between family members are profoundly affected by eating disorders. Eating disorders put strain on every family member, significant others, and loved ones in a unique way. Watching loved ones do such harm to themselves leaved those affected feeling powerless and helpless. I often hear family members describe their experience as constantly feeling like they are walking on eggshells, unable to understand, being pushed away, overwhelmed and scared, angry, or even guilty over seeing their loved one in so much pain. Everyone needs support, everyone needs to be educated, everyone deserves to be heard and acknowledged. At times, I have seen a great deal of initial willingness from the family when the treatment recommendation includes some form of family therapy. However, this willingness often turns to resistance once the family has received some education and is encouraged to do some deeper therapeutic work. However, we must tell that family, that an eating disorder is a family problem and not a sick child problem. Everyone needs and deserves support, nurturing and validation.

A trained therapist also facilitates family therapy. Family therapy involves members of an immediate or extended family. A careful assessment of the entire family, meaning the identified patient, his or her parents and siblings, and any other significant members of the patient's family. The family therapist will also obtain a thorough development history, including emotional, social, and physical development. Family therapy provides a forum where each family member can become educated about the complexities of this disease. The most common form of family therapy used is based on family systems theory. The family systems model shows how family member plays a part in the whole system. It emphasizes factors such as family roles, relationships, and communication patterns. This approach accepts the family itself as the patient, with the presenting member, the patient, viewed as a sign of family psychopathology. Many therapists may recommend an additional therapist to facilitate family therapy if they assess that it is in the best interest of the client. This may be helpful for the initial therapeutic relationship to remain safe, objective, and trusting. Early in recovery, family members and significant others may also need a safe place to communicate their own concerns and needs without the sufferer being present.

The Maudsley family-based outpatient treatment for anorexia nervosa is a promising treatment approach for adolescents. The Maudsley approach can mostly be construed as an intensive outpatient treatment where parents play an active and positive role in order to help restore their child's weight to normal levels expected given their adolescent's age and height; hand the control over eating back to the adolescent, and; encourage normal adolescent development through an in-depth discussion of these crucial developmental issues as they pertain to their child.[54] To learn more about Maudsley treatment approach, visit www.maudsleyparents.org.

Group Therapy

A small group of thoughtful people can change the world. Indeed, it's the only thing that ever has.

-Margaret Mead

Group therapy offers multiple relationships to assist the individual in growth and problem solving. Each type of group has a different orientation with a different focus and format.

The number of sessions in group therapy depends upon the group's makeup, goals, and setting. Certain groups are more appropriate for individuals at different stages in their recovery. Any member of the treatment team as well as other specialized treatment professionals may facilitate specific groups. Some examples of different topics for group therapy utilized in eating disorder treatment programs include:

1. Body image

2. CBT

3. Affirmations

4. Motivational goal setting

5. Life story

6. Guided imagery

7. Art therapy

8. Daily journal

9. Family dynamics

10. Healthy sexuality

11. Nutritional education

12. Meal support groups

13. Experiential Eating

14. DBT (mindfulness, emotional regulation, interpersonal effectiveness, and distress tolerance)

15. Yoga

16. Life tools

17. Drama therapy

18. Coping skills

19. Movement therapy

20. Assertiveness training

21. Reading/Discussion/Letter Writing

22. Spirituality

23. Addictions

24. Community meetings

25. Healthy relationships

YALOM – Therapeutic Factors

Dr. Irvin Yalom in his book *The Theory and Practice of Group Therapy*[106] identifies 11 "curative factors" or "therapeutic factors" that are the "primary agents of change" in group therapy. Yalom refers to these therapeutic factors as an intricate interplay of human experience. Each of the therapeutic factors serves their own unique purpose and facilitates psychological change in ways that individual therapy cannot. The therapeutic factors are listed below along with an explanation of their importance in the treatment of eating disorders.

1. **Instillation of hope** - The group facilitator should help a client have faith and feel optimistic that change and resolution are possible. This factor is one that may need to be continually reinforced, especially because is so much despair and isolation that occurs with eating disorders. This is especially true during the early stages of recovery.

Example: In the majority of groups I have facilitated, there was almost always a group member who had been further along in their recovery who shared their movement from despair to hope. This has most definitely been extremely beneficial time and time again.

2. **Universality** - This factor helps an individual know that they are not alone and isolated with unique psychological issues.

   Example: It is such a critical therapeutic factor when facilitating eating disorder groups, since secrecy has been such a strong isolating factor. Secrecy and social isolation are common themes with eating disorders. I have watched clients encountering others who have suffered similar violations and deep feelings of shame, guilt, and rage. I have seen this be so useful in helping to relieve the stigma that goes along with an eating disorder.

3. **Imparting of information** - This is also known as psychoeducating clients. Yalom[106] says that "didactic instruction is used to transfer information, alter sabotaging thought patterns and explain the process of illness...Direct advice which provides systematic, operationalized instruction or a series of alternative suggestions on how to reach a goal is most effective.[106] Education on all aspects of eating disorders including the physical, emotional, spiritual, and psychological impact on oneself and others are just a few topics of didactic instruction. This type of instruction has shown itself to be effective for teaching mindfulness stress reduction and relapse prevention.

4. **Altruism** - The act of giving without expecting anything in return is the meaning of altruism. Altruism is so critical to note because another common theme with

eating disorders is seeing oneself as a burden, and not believing one has anything to offer. Learning to give and receive graciously has such enormous healing power.

Example: So often, those suffering from eating disorders describe being "so in my head" to the point that they are unable to engage in random acts of kindness. This becomes a problem because an eating disorder sufferer is usually an individual who is genuinely king, caring, and giving by nature. With that being said, if an individual is so locked in an eating disorder and unable to engage in random acts of kindness then she is actually going against her true authentic self. This can inevitably lead to increased self-judgment, depression, and self-criticism. This is most often an unconscious process. Therefore, this is an extremely important therapeutic factor. I have seen clients even leave on a two week to six month sabbatical to practice the act of altruism, who have come back with a sense of fulfillment and peace.

5. **Corrective recapitulation of primary family group** - The relationships with other group members can give clients a chance to correctively relive early family conflicts, and relationships that inhibited growth.

   Example: competitiveness between group members can often be a factor indicative of sibling rivalry. The re-enactment of parent-child dynamics, splitting amongst group leaders, and the recapitulation of the good parent and the bad parent is often very apparent in my experience.

6. **Development of socializing techniques** - Social learning, or the development of basic social skills, is a therapeutic outcome that occurs in all therapy groups. Yalom acknowledged that for individuals lacking intimate

relationships, the group often represents the first opportunity for accurate interpersonal feedback."[106]

Example: since the individual suffering from an eating disorder is experiencing so much sadness, and an inconsolable loneliness, group therapy provides a rich opportunity for members to learn how they contribute to their own isolation and loneliness. I have also found it fascinating to watch clients begin to understand the actual incongruence between what they intend to say and the actual impact they have on others.

7. **Imitative behavior** - Much like the development of socializing techniques, by imitating the behavior of the therapist and other group members, the client can explore and begin to establish more of a stable unique sense of self.

Example: I can see where imitative behavior can be imperative to learning yet, I can also see where the therapist must keep a close eye. For example, in a homogeneous group of addicts and eating disorder sufferers, the individual almost inevitably lacks a stable sense of self. Imitative behavior is extremely beneficial as long as it stays separate from idealized behavior and the behaviors being imitated are healthy ones.

8. **Interpersonal learning** - These skills, when generalized into the world at large, can help clients establish interpersonal effectiveness. Hendrix (1998) describes the concept of interpersonal learning quite well: "We are born in a relationship, we are wounded in a relationship, and we can be healed within a relationship. Indeed, we cannot be fully healed outside of a relationship." [41]

Example: I reflect back and think about how often I have heard and continue to hear that "you shouldn't care what anyone thinks of you," or "I don't care what anyone thinks about me." Oftentimes, I have seen that these statements are looked upon with envy. One may believe that it is actually a sign of strength to not care what others think and a sign of weakness when one places too much emphasis on what others believe. I believe this is actually a very dangerous belief and as much as I know it is a defense, it usually only exacerbates the presenting symptoms. One cannot live in a plastic bubble. To create a solid sense of self, it is critical to integrate how one sees self, how one wants others to see them, and how they are actually perceived by others. I think about how many clients make assumptions or utilize mind reading to feed their self-loathing thoughts, already "knowing" what "everyone" thinks and feels about them. Interpersonal learning is an especially important factor amongst those in recovery.

9. **Catharsis** - A therapeutic factor that occurs when an individual can express their deep emotional feelings, and can experience a release and healing. A powerful cathartic experience comes from one having an intense emotional release and it has an even greater impact when there is strong group cohesiveness.

    Example: Once of my philosophies is quite simple: You must feel to heal....

10. **Existential factors** - Recognition of the basic features of existence through sharing with others (e.g., ultimate aloneness, ultimate death, ultimate responsibility for our own actions.) Existentialism is a psychological and philosophical theory that recognizes that life can be unfair and unjust at times, that there is no escape from pain, that no matter how close we get to other individuals we are ultimately alone, and that there is

no escape from the inevitability of death. Living in fear of these outcomes cause great suffering.

Example: This is an area where I often see great suffering. It can be incredibly frightening to face these inevitable life truths. I often see clients express great discomfort, anxiety, and even heightened resistance when asked to identify and explore their thoughts and feelings around these existential topics. This often intense angst that surrounds facing these fears can be more debilitating than one knows. The eating disorder may provide a distraction, a false sense of comfort or control, or even a means to communicate their fears of the unknown. Yet, even when the client is educated about how facing these fears can result in a great sense of freedom and even increased courage to let go of one's eating disorder, it is often initially met with resistance. This is also about a connection to something bigger than ourselves and may even force the client to examine one's spiritual beliefs and faith. Eating disorders are a strong and powerful tool to use to fill, discard, or even relieve that void. Groups provide a safe atmosphere to begin to explore these topics, especially when a client finds they are not alone.

11. **Group cohesiveness** - This is a primary factor and allows members to believe that they belong somewhere, that they value the group, and that they feel valued and supported by the other members.

Example: I have seen much power in this factor. When a group becomes cohesive, so many wonderful things emerge. Just to begin with, members start to look forward to coming to group. Treatment may actually become "sometimes even kind of fun." Due to group cohesiveness I have seen laughter, tears, silliness, courage, and hope.

Case Vignette Background Information
-Interplay of Yalom's Therapeutic Factors-

An actual clinical vignette will illustrate the interplay of these therapeutic factors. The names, ages, and some other criteria of these clients are fictional in nature. This particular group met several times a week in a partial hospitalization outpatient program for the treatment of eating disorders. Before presenting this vignette I will provide you with some relevant background information for each for the women presented.

Background Information

Jennifer is a 23-year-old female who has been hospitalized on numerous occasions for anorexia, bulimia, depression, and cutting. Jennifer was sexually abused by her father for most of her childhood and early adolescence. Her mother continues to live in denial to the point where Jennifer often questions her own reality. Jennifer has a great deal of resistance towards letting go of her self-destructive behaviors. She has poor interpersonal skills, often tends to disconnect, speaks very softly, and utilizes isolation as a defense. She is an extreme perfectionist, very intelligent, has great difficulty receiving compliments, and experiences continual shame and guilt. I will classify Jennifer as the "silent" and the "boring" client. Yalom[106] indicates that "some are silent for fear of being regarded as weak, insipid, or mawkish" and this definitely fits Jennifer. Yalom[106] describes the "boring client as one who is massively inhibited, who lacks spontaneity, and who never takes risks."

Samantha is a 26-year-old female who has also had numerous hospitalizations for anorexia and bulimia, as well as individual therapy on and off for the past 12 years. She fluctuates between extreme loves and hate in all her relationships, displays constant splitting, and blames everyone else for abandoning her. She is the middle child of six, lost her mother to cancer when she was 17, and has also been diagnosed at different times with Bipolar Disorder and Borderline Personality Disorder. Samantha is an actress and dancer, and presents herself as very provocative and yet is extremely defensive and narcissistic. Let us refer to Samantha as both "The Borderline Client" and "The Narcissistic Client." Yalom[106] states that "therapy groups offer the borderline individual containment, emotional support, and interpersonal learning while demanding personal accountability" which is crucial for Samantha's treatment.

Liz is a 17-year-old female who came into the treatment program after recently having been discharged from a drug rehabilitation center. Liz is very friendly, is a caretaker, avoids conflict, yet is emotionally unstable and manipulative. Liz grew up as an only child in a family with an alcoholic mother, who displayed bipolar and narcissistic traits, and an absent father. Liz took on the family role of the parentifed child, where the child is inappropriately given the role of meeting the emotional or physical needs of the parent or of the other children. As the parentifed child, Liz will protect her mother at all costs, and is experiencing enormous guilt that she is receiving treatment. Liz also carries a great deal of repressed anger.

Case Vignette
-Interplay of Yalom's Therapeutic Factors-

Samantha, the narcissistic and borderline client, had been very loving and consoling to Jennifer, the silent and boring client, throughout the time they had both been members of the group. Although, the majority of this "love and support" from Samantha to Jennifer normally took place right before the group began, after the close of group, or during the short breaks before group. It had appeared that this relationship lacked reciprocity and allowed Samantha to remain narcissistic and Jennifer to remain silent. However, one group proved to be drastically different. Samantha began this group with a hostile attack on Jennifer. She stated that she was so sick and tired of disclosing so much, taking risks in being vulnerable with others, and constantly watching Jennifer be silent, almost invisible, and never sharing anything about herself. Each of the group members responded differently, either immediately protecting Jennifer, saying nothing, or looking to me as the group leader to step in to diffuse any discomfort. Either way, the dialog, both silent or verbal, that was going on about her or around her, was contributing to keeping Jennifer invisible and in a preverbal state.

It had been continually clear that the group members were apprehensiveness to speak directly to Samantha about her aggressive behavior. Yet, out of nowhere Liz suddenly became very angry directly with Samantha for the aggressive manner in which she addressed Jennifer. This was the first time Liz had ever expressed strong negative affect in this group. It was no coincidence that Samantha became the culprit of the anger Liz had such difficulty expressing. The feelings Liz was experiencing were very similar to the emotions she had towards her own mother. In that moment, however, Liz was no longer able or willing to disguise or repress her emotions.

Samantha was taken aback as it was extremely rare for her to allow herself to be the recipient of anger. She initially became very defensive towards Liz, and actually got up and left the room. One of the other group members agreed to go out and check on her safety, and to nurture her frantic efforts to avoid real or imagined abandonment. It was at this point that Jennifer began to apologize stating, "I'm sorry Liz, this is all my fault." Simultaneously, Liz also became frightened and apologetic. One of the other experienced group members stated, "Neither of you needs to apologize. Thank you, this is wonderful, it is so good to get to really hear from you both."

Samantha did finally return to group after she had calmed down and she did apologize to both Liz and Jennifer. Samantha showed up late for the next group session and acted out in many other ways as well. Ultimately, Samantha did some excellent work during this particular group experience. Liz and Jennifer began to form a friendship that still continues to this day.

Case Vignette Explanation
-Interplay of Yalom's Therapeutic Factors-

The style of my intervention began by observing Jennifer's reception of the information imparted to her by Samantha. Due to Jennifer's fragile sense of self, I engaged in repeated process checks with Jennifer to monitor her ability to tolerate this amount of stimulation, while keeping in mind the defensive and at times aggressive nature of Samantha. I knew that this issue was far too important to be left unexplored. Being aware of the <u>group cohesiveness</u>, the amount of time the group had been together, the additional support through individual therapy both women were receiving, the continual small doses of addressing Jennifer's silence and Samantha's unpredictability, and the timing and instinct, I believed it was just the right opportunity for continued process exploration.

<u>Universality</u> was at play in helping these young women to learn that they are not so different than others. It was very powerful for these women to see they are not alone in their shame and stigma, especially since these factors greatly contribute to their social isolation. All three of these women experience anger. Jennifer turns hers inward, Liz disconnects from it entirely, and Samantha purges her anger, similar to the purging of her food, outwards towards others. Yet, these women all have an extremely fragile sense of self, feel unappreciated, misunderstood, and overlooked by all those living around them. Their anger (as well as other factors) serves them as a way to avoid emotional intimacy, continue to feel isolated, lack close friendships, and feeds their belief that no one will ever truly understand them. Staying in the here-and-now with heightened awareness of the extreme discomfort of the group members, I helped the clients be more receptive by utilizing empathy and reflective listening. This helped to reduce the tension to a tolerable level for the group to reconnect.

For all group members, <u>altruism</u> is extremely important, but for sake of discussion, this therapeutic factor was highly significant for Jennifer. Paradoxically, Jennifer saw her silence and being "invisible" as an altruistic behavior because of her deep rooted belief that she was undeserving of taking up space or having a voice. She experienced her silence as a selfless attribute, as a benefit to others, because it was her way to avoid potential or further conflict. Jennifer needed to see that she had something to give, such as compassion, genuine kindness, and empathy, and that others greatly benefit from these unconditional gifts. When Jennifer actually did begin to use her voice in group and clearly saw the other members benefit from her input, she was increasingly able to engage in altruistic behaviors, thus increasing self-esteem. The positive responses Jennifer received when she spoke, also challenged her old belief that silence was a selfless attribute. This would prove to be a great accomplishment to her continued growth and helped to initially decrease her fears of social eating. Yalom made a statement in the <u>existential factors</u> section of the book that is quite applicable to Jennifer. He said, "Being useful to someone else drew her out of morbid self-absorption and provided her with a sense of purpose and meaning."[106] Due to her history of being sexually abused by her father and the lack of protection she received from her mother, it was so incredible for Jennifer to see that she was useful to others because of who she is and because of the value in her feedback.

Liz experienced a <u>corrective emotional experience</u> of her primary family group when she was able to verbalize that she was continually afraid of upsetting Samantha. Remember, Liz was the parentified child and that her mother was both a drug addict and was diagnosed with bipolar disorder. Liz was continually fearful of upsetting her mother, protected her at all costs, and therefore, held all of her emotions in. She utilized catastrophizing as a defense because she had such a deep belief that her expression of anger could actually cause her mother to fall apart, and that in the end she would be responsible for her mother's death. Yet, even with her expression of anger towards someone who had many similar traits as her mother, no catastrophe actually occurred. Although Samantha did respond to Liz with defensiveness and actually left the room-which may have actually reinforced her distorted beliefs-Samantha did come back after she received this high level of anger from Liz, and she actually apologized for her aggression. This was truly a <u>catharsis</u> for Liz, and the beginning of her introspective work. Liz began to see that her avoidance of anger had been truly irrational, and was very dangerous for her well-being. This was also a cathartic moment for Samantha because her intense fear of abandonment proved to be false. The group was still there, and slowly began working on giving and receiving more authenticity.

In regards to <u>interpersonal learning,</u> these young women began to gain insight and to explore what their behavior was like through feedback. This feedback provided information on how their behavior made others feel. Samantha's tendency was to be unaware of both her interpersonal impact and of the response of others to her. This is an area she continued to have difficulty with. Role-play was a very useful therapeutic tool for Samantha to teach the difference between assertive and aggressive forms of communication. Jennifer was given feedback that was very inviting. A couple of group members provided empathic attunement, and with kindness and love they shared how much they would value her input but, were often hesitant to help bring her into greater group involvement. Jennifer was actually able to verbalize how difficult it was for her to ask for help, and how she often felt like such a burden. Liz then shared that she had the same experience as Jennifer when it came to asking for help. At that point, I utilized didactic instruction to help both Liz and Jennifer to identify internal and external bodily cues that indicate they are experiencing an emotional response to material being discussed. The group members shared their own cues to assist both women. To help Jennifer take more personal responsibility, she and the group leader came up with a signal she could initially use if she was experiencing any affective experience. Over the next couple of months, Jennifer became able to engage in self-disclosure and to give feedback at least one time every group session. She also began to see clearly the similarity between how her behaviors that contribute to her isolation in group mimic her behaviors in her outside interpersonal relationships. Imparting information regarding healthy communication and emotional regulation was also very valuable, especially for Liz.

This case vignette clearly shows the incredible work that can be accomplished in group therapy. At times, it can be exhausting and exhilarating all within the same group. I have continued to see that these ever so present therapeutic factors provide continual lessons of life. They teach us how to regulate our emotions, how to tolerate discomfort and frustration, and how to create and maintain healthy relationships. Beyond the actual "eating disorder behaviors," this is a great deal of what recovery from an eating disorder is about.

Twelve-Step Model of Treatment

Yesterday is history, tomorrow's a
mystery, and today is a gift.
-12 step fellowship recovery quotes

Are eating disorders addictions? Consider the core features of addictions. The American Society of Addiction Medicine has this definition for addiction: characterized by impairment in behavioral control, craving, inability to consistently abstain, and diminished recognition of significant problems with one's behaviors and interpersonal relationships. In regards to viewing an eating disorder through the addictions model, many professionals believe complete recovery from an eating disorder is attainable. The addictions model views an individual as always being "recovering" versus "recovered." Some believe that the mindset of always being "recovering" can contribute to a belief system that leaves room for relapse, which can be detrimental for eating disorder sufferers.

The twelve-step model of treatment began with Alcoholics Anonymous (AA).[1] The 12-step approach can help instill hope and faith for recovery, give women a common language for discussing spirituality, provide a concrete action plan for using one's faith in recovery, and offer a support network that can help prevent relapse.[83] As summarized by the American Psychological Association, the components of the program, which differ but are also a synopsis, from the specific 12 steps and traditions, include:

- Admitting that one cannot control one's addiction compulsive behaviors

- Utilizing spirituality as a way of gaining strength

- Examining past errors with the help of a sponsor

- Making amends for these errors

- Learning to live a new recovery-oriented life

- Helping others that suffer from the same addictions or compulsions.

There are two primary fellowships that serve people with eating disorders: Overeaters Anonymous (OA) and Eating Disorders Anonymous (EDA). These groups have numerous benefits. They provide support in a caring environment and help reduce feelings of shame around use of eating disorder symptoms and behaviors. A benefit of twelve step programs is that there are no dues or fees for membership. These programs are entirely self-supporting through literature sales and member contributions. In addition, they do not solicit or accept outside contributions. Meetings are also readily available throughout most communities. There is additional support through the sense of community created as well as through the programs' sponsors who work closely with individuals, guiding and helping one work through the twelve steps.

Overeater's Anonymous (OA)

The smartest thing an OA member can say, is help me.

-*Overeaters Anonymous*

Overeater's Anonymous (OA) is a fellowship of individuals who through shared experience, strength and hope are recovering from compulsive overeating and to carry this message of recovery to those who still suffer.[75] Even though symptoms may vary, OA claims that there is a shared bond: we are powerless over food and our lives are unmanageable.

Eating Disorders Anonymous (EDA)

*The principles embodied in the 12 steps of EDA
include--Honesty, Equality, Accountability, Love,
Trust, and Humility (Health: the EDA motto)*
-Eating Disorders Anonymous

A newer twelve-step program focused on eating disorder recovery is known as Eating Disorders Anonymous (EDA). Eating Disorders Anonymous is a fellowship of individuals (founded in February 2000 by members of Alcoholics Anonymous in Phoenix) who share their experience, strength and hope with each other that they may solve their common problems and help others to recover from their eating disorders. The only requirement for membership is a desire to recover from an eating disorder. The meetings are focused on helping people live without obsessing about food, weight, and body image. They define recovery as "gaining" or regaining the power to see our options to make careful choices in our lives. Many professionals who treat eating disorders prefer this model as it embraces the steps of AA for recovery but is not based on the addiction model. Rather than suggesting abstinence as a way to recovery, which is what OA does, it instead focuses on balance.

Twelve-step used as an adjunct to other treatment can be very beneficial. Many individuals indicate that meetings provide support in a safe and non-judgmental environment. Meetings are also a place where they can share what others may not understand. These factors alone can help the process of healing. Most importantly, each being needs to be viewed as a unique individual and recovery support needs are equally unique. Everyone deserves and needs to explore treatment options that work best for them. I encourage all individuals to continue to explore their needs and options that best fit their support needs throughout treatment.

We all need people in our recovery. For some who are in recovery from eating disorders, achieving a twelve step eating disorders focused home group, or fellowship has been a saving grace. Others have found it to be too triggering and confusing: these express difficulty connecting to the spiritual principals, especially that of a higher power. So again, even if it does not work or seem like a match early on in your recovery; I encourage each client to stay open minded, take a chance to revisit adjunctive, and spiritually based models as they move further in recovery. Remember, flexibility is an important component to recovery.

Complementary and Alternative Therapies

Alternative therapies tend to take a holistic approach-treating the entirety of an individual. The National Center for Complementary and Alternative Medicine (NCCAM)[68] defines complementary and alternative medicine as a group of diverse medical and health care systems, practices, and products that are not generally considered part of conventional medicine. A common function of these approaches is using focused imagery in a relaxed state of mind. Anyone interested in complementary and alternative therapies for the treatment of eating disorders should receive medical clearance before undergoing any therapy.

Common **alternative therapies** are most often used adjunctively with the more traditional and conventional treatment approaches. Mind and body practices focus on the interactions among the brain, mind, body, and behavior, with the intent to use the mind to affect physical functioning and promote health. Some of the more common examples of mind and body practices include:

Acupuncture

Acupuncture is a traditional Chinese treatment, based on the belief that our bodies have energy meridians or channels, and that ill health, both physical and psychological, results from blockages or imbalances in these channels. Acupuncture is a treatment in which small needles are inserted into the skin at specific points to relieve pain and promote healing. This is known to help balance the energy in the body. Acupuncture can help with the physical symptoms of an eating disorder. It can be used to ease digestive and GI symptoms including bloating and constipation. It can also help improve the functioning of the digestive system.

Meditation

There are essentially two forms of meditation: insight and concentration. Mindfulness is considered insight mediation since it brings full attention to the body and mind in the present moment without trying to alter or manipulate the experience. Whatever is occurring in the body (sights, sounds, smells, tastes, sensations) or mind, the task is simply to observe its ever-changing nature. Put in even simpler terms, mindfulness consists of cultivating awareness of the mind and body and living in the here and now.

In concentration meditation, the focus is on concepts, images, or a mantra. This can also be referred to as *guided imagery* or visualization. It is a technique in which the individual is directed by a person (either in person or by using a pre-recorded voice) to relax and envision certain images and scenes to promote relaxation and create a sense of tranquility. With concentration meditation, you become one with the object of focus, whereas with insight meditation you begin to see the ever-changing nature of body and mind. Both are methods of suspending thought and directing attention in a calm and focused manner. Daily meditations, which include recovery-based intentions, are extremely beneficial.

Motivating eating disorder sufferers to practice meditation is often a challenge, at least initially. Many sufferers have a preconceived notion about meditation and fear tells them that there is no way they will be able to "do it." Yet, due to constant chatter that goes on in the mind of an eating disorder sufferer, meditation may be an invaluable prescription. Meditation can also help one to develop a more balanced relationship within oneself, one's eating, and one's body.

Massage

Massage is a manipulative and body-based practice that has long been utilized to produce emotional release, improve mood, help circulation,and increase relaxation. Studies shows that people with body image disturbances have often been deprived of nurturing touch or have been violated with the use of touch. To these individuals, massage can seem frightening. I have heard many state,"I don't want anyone touching my body," only to learn that when touch is nurturing, safe, loving, without judgment and expectations, the entire experience can be healing. This may take time, but again it is of heightened importance to work with someone who has knowledge and experience working with eating disorders and trauma.

Biofeedback

Biofeedback is a method of monitoring minute metabolic changes in one's own body with the aid of sensitive machines. Individuals learn to make subtle adjustments to move towards a more balanced internal state by consciously visualizing, relaxing, or imagining while observing light, sound, or metered feedback.

Aromatherapy

Aromatherapy is the therapeutic use of essential oils extracted from roots, stems, leaves, bark, flowers or other parts of a plant used to achieve health and vitality. Some of the specific functions of aromatherapy include pain relief, mood enhancement, reduction of anxiety and insomnia, and increased cognitive function. The inhaled aroma from these essential oils, the pure essence of the plant, is widely believed to stimulate brain function and influence physical, emotional, and mental health. Essential oils can also be applied directly to the skin, where they travel through the bloodstream to support whole body healing.

Although essential oils have been utilized for centuries, there is minimal scientific evidence regarding the safety and effectiveness of aromatherapy. However, many individuals clearly experience benefits from the use of aromatherapy. While there are currently no boards that certify or license aromatherapists in the United States, many are trained in some other form of therapy, such as massage or chiropractic, and include aromatherapy in their practice.

Homeopathy

Homeopathy, also known as *homeopathic medicine*, is the therapeutic use of small doses of medicines which stimulate the body's natural defense systems. The intention is to re-balance the body. Homeopathic remedies are highly diluted substances that are extracted from substances that come from animal, plant, or minerals. Qualified homeopaths should be registered with the Society of Homeopaths.

Experiential Therapies

These types of therapies are meant to increase your awareness of being in the present moment. Practices that help you focus on your moment-by-moment thoughts, feelings, and sensations will anchor you in the present and help you to reconnect to yourself on every level. These types of therapies are incredibly powerful to utilize in conjunction with traditional therapies.

Because of the power of experiential therapies, it is best if the therapist is trained in working with eating disorders. There is much trauma that often co-exists with eating disorders and it is believed that trauma memories, reactions to life's threatening experiences, can be stored and recorded in the body. Negative, frightening, and unpleasant memories and sensations can easily be accessed without the knowledge that this can occur. That can be extremely confusing and frightening. So, if this occurs when the therapist lacks the tools to help provide containment, understanding, and reassurance, it can in fact be a re-traumatizing experience. The point is, that these are amazing and powerful tools to promote healing, and are even more so when employed in conjunction with the multi-disciplinary team.

Yoga

The various styles of yoga used for health purposes typically combine physical postures, breathing techniques, and meditation or relaxation. Yoga can be an effective tool to restore the imbalances in both the body and the mind that occur with eating disorders. Yoga has a profound ability to balance the emotions and has been shown to help elevate mood, to relieve anxiety and to promote equanimity, which is a calm, clear and focused mind.

Dance/Movement Therapy (DMT)

DMT uses body sensations and body movement as a source of healing. It is important for those suffering from eating disorders to learn how to use their bodies, as a positive tool for self-expression. Connecting to the power and beauty of the body is an amazing experience. Dance movement therapists believe this concept makes perfect sense because the body is the battleground where the eating disorder occurs. DMT helps one to gain a more solid sense of body boundaries and personal space. Dance Movement therapists must have a Master's degree and meet other requirements set by their professional organization, The American Dance Therapy Association.

Art Therapy

Art therapy helps one to use numerous means of artistic expression. So many have difficulty expressing themselves through their words and the power of the hands can be extremely healing. There are so many materials to be used from the simple sketchpad, to the use of chalks, clay, and paint, to mosaic materials, anything to everything. Creating an object to represent various parts of one's self and even utilizing visualization can work as the catalyst to explore so many aspects of self. If art therapy is done with someone who is trained and understands how to help you find the meanings and interpretations, the experience is that much more enhanced. It would be best to work with a Registered Art Therapist (ATR) who has training in working with eating disorder clients.

Music Therapy

Music therapy promotes healing through an expressive form without having to talk. This type of therapy is extremely powerful as it can activate such a wide array of emotions. Listening to music, playing music, writing music stimulates the senses and can help to elevate mood, express oneself in ways never thought possible, and self-soothe. Exploring new sounds and listening to music you may have never listened to while you were locked in your eating disorder can help with learning distress tolerance skills and how to use music to bring light instead of reaffirming darkness. These factors will only enhance successful recovery. The American Music Therapy Association sets the education and clinical training standards for music therapists.

———6———

LEVELS OF CARE FOR TREATMENT

Take the first step in faith. You don't have to see
the whole staircase, just take the first step.

-Martin Luther King

As discussed previously, treatment from an Eating Disorder may take place in numerous types of treatment settings. You will learn in the next chapter how to determine the appropriate Level of Care by careful examination of the Guidelines.

Outpatient Treatment

The most unstructured treatment takes place on an Outpatient basis. This type of treatment may involve a patient receiving individual therapy once or twice a week, meeting with a Registered Dietitian one time a week, and if necessary, working with a Primary Care Physician or Pediatrician. These doctors will send the patient out for the necessary lab work. Other treatment professionals include specialists in other areas, such as a dentist for the patient who suffers from bulimia Nervosa, an OB/GYN for female concerns, a cardiologist for additional medical concerns. In addition, the patient may be given outside referrals to increase support system. Some of these referrals, which were discussed in the previous chapter, include 12 step programs, community support groups, and whatever else may be necessary. The patient receiving treatment at this level of care is functioning normally, with possibly a little impairment in areas of interpersonal relationships, and vocational, or educational functioning. If at any time a patient's symptoms become exacerbated and her level of functioning seems to begin to deteriorate, and she appears to need more support, the patient will most likely be referred to a higher level of care.

Intensive Outpatient Program (IOP)

An Intensive Outpatient Program (IOP), formally identified as Day Treatment Program (DTP), is a structured program, which most often includes individual therapy, group therapy, and nutritional support with a Registered Dietitian. An IOP program can range from three to six days a week for three to four hours a day. This level of care is appropriate for an individual whose eating disorder is not being contained at a lower level of care, and requires increased support and structure. Patients may also enter this level of care as a step-down from a higher level of care, Partial Hospitalization, Residential Treatment, or an Inpatient Setting. This structure will help the patient integrate more into his or her daily life. The following criteria may determine this level of care:

A. Medical Stability

1. Daily monitoring or medical needs is not necessary.

B. Psychiatric/Psychological Stability

1. Symptoms are still present, yet the patient is able to participate in a normal capacity in daily functioning in their social, vocational, and educational environment.

2. Psychological distress is present and significant, but not debilitating.

Partial Hospitalization Program (PHP)

A Partial Hospitalization Program (PHP) is a structured five to six day per week Outpatient Program. The program typically consists of an eight-hour day Monday through Friday along with a three to five hour day on Saturday. As with IOP, there is a program designed for both the adult and adolescent patient. An individual may enter this level of care directly from outpatient treatment or an Intensive Outpatient Program (IOP) as they require intensive support and structure. This level of care is also appropriate as a step-down from a higher level of care, namely, a Residential or Inpatient Treatment setting. The purpose of a Partial Hospitalization Program is to help individuals gain awareness and work through their eating disorder and other related disorders in a highly structured outpatient treatment setting while integrating their growth and new recovery with their outside environment. The following criteria may help determine this level of care:

A. Medical Stability

1. Eating Disorder medical concerns may impair functioning without acute risk.

B. Psychiatric/Psychological Stability

1. Interpersonal relationships are gravely affected and there is an inability to function in their outside environment.

2. Severely restricting food, daily bingeing, purging, excessive exercise, and other excessive weight control behaviors.

A program at the PHP level of care will most likely involve:

1. Vitals Daily

2. Psychiatric Follow-Ups (1-3 times a week)

3. Individual Therapy (1-2 times a week)

4. Family Therapy and a Multi-Family Support Group

5. Nutritional and Exercise Counseling by a Registered Dietitian up to two times a week.

6. Group Therapy

7. Eating two meals a day with the other individuals in treatment.

Residential Treatment

Residential treatment is a 24-hour-a-day live-in facility that provides around the clock intensive supervision and extensive treatment. This intensive supervision and support are still needed to help the sufferer stop self-destructive eating disorder behaviors that may still remain out of control. Specialized psychological intervention is more intensive then what is available in the majority of inpatient treatment settings. This is especially due to the fact, that an Inpatient level of care is focused on medical stabilization, usually short-term and about crisis stabilization. Residential treatment programs may be located in medical hospitals or exist separately on home-like grounds or estates. The criteria below are typical for treatment at this level of care:

A. Medical Stability

    1. Patient is medically stable and requires no intensive medical intervention.

B. Psychiatric/Psychological Stability

    1. Patient is psychiatrically impaired.

    2. Patient is unable to respond to Partial Hospitalization or Outpatient treatment.

Inpatient Treatment

Inpatient treatment is 24-hour-care which can be in a hospital setting or a psychiatric facility. Again, it is usually a short-term stay and is focused on crisis stabilization. An inpatient setting is used to treat medical complications that have arisen as a result of an eating disorder. The criteria for a patient who requires an <u>Inpatient</u> level of care demonstrates medical instability pursuant to the following:

A. Medical Stability

    1. Unstable or depressed vital signs.

    2. Laboratory findings present an acute health risk.

    3. Complications due to coexisting medical problems such as diabetes.

B. Psychiatric/Psychological Stability

    1. Rapidly worsening symptoms.

    2. Suicidal and unable to contract for safety.

The decision to receive treatment for an eating disorder is often a frightening and overwhelming process. However, once a client has readily agreed to receive treatment, it is beneficial to move as quickly as possible before the "Eating Disorder Mind" takes control again. If a friend or loved one is suffering from an eating disorder, it is important to begin becoming knowledgeable of the many options available.

The intensity and duration of treatment depends on numerous factors including insurance coverage limits and ability to pay for treatment, severity and duration of the disorder, mental health status, and coexisting medical or psychological disorders. A crucial step in choosing the best treatment center, based on the unique needs of each particular individual, is to become educated about and to understand eating disorder treatment programs and the levels of care that are available. A health care professional or a treatment team, if one is already in place, can help one understand the difference between the intensity and structure of these various levels of care.

Once an individual has made a decision to enter treatment, it is best to have the patient be as involved as possible in becoming educated on the treatment options, including various levels of care. The more a patient is involved in this decision-making process, the more likely they are to be invested in their own recovery. An individual suffering from an eating disorder already has difficulty identifying and expressing their needs, lacks assertiveness skills, struggles with trusting one's decision-making abilities, and using one's voice. So, the eating disorder sufferer's involvement in this decision-making process is an opportunity to begin engaging in one's growth.

7

LEVEL OF CARE TREATMENT GUIDELINES

The "Level of Care Guidelines for Patients with Eating Disorders" were formulated and noted in *The Practice Guidelines for the Treatment of Patients with Eating Disorders.*[5,105] These guidelines are extremely useful and relevant in helping to determine what level of care the patient may require. Of course, consultation with other professionals is always beneficial and is in the best interest of the patient. These guidelines include outpatient care, intensive outpatient care, Partial Hospitalization (Full-Day Outpatient Care), Residential Treatment, and Inpatient Hospitalization. In general, a given level of care should be considered for patients who meet one or more criteria for a particular level. The guidelines are not absolutes, however, and their application requires physician judgment.[53] In addition, the level of care must be continually assessed throughout the treatment of an eating disorder patient because their treatment needs may change over time.

There are many factors to take into account when making appropriate level of care decisions. The three factors that are of most importance are *medical status, suicidality, and weight as percentage of healthy body weight.*

Medical Status This factor alone can determine the need for a higher level of care for treatment of a patient with an eating disorder. It is in the best interest of the patient and the therapist for the patient to receive medical clearance from a physician even at the outpatient level of care. This clearance can also serve as a baseline as you continue treatment.

Suicidality If a patient discloses any suicidal thoughts, the professional must explore lethality, intent, means, and specificity. If it is determined that suicidality is present, a higher level of care may be necessary depending on the estimated level of risk. It is imperative that any current or prior suicidal ideation or history of attempts be assessed when treating an eating disorder patient. Inpatient hospitalization may be necessary if a patient discloses a specific plan with high lethality or intent. Determining suicide risk is a complex clinical judgment, as is determining the most appropriate treatment setting for a patient at risk for suicide. Relevant factors to consider are the patient's concurrent medical condition, psychosis, substance use, other psychiatric symptoms or syndromes, psychosocial supports, past suicidal behaviors, treatment adherence, and the quality of existing physician-patient relationships. These factors are described in greater detail in the APA's *Practice Guideline for the Assessment and Treatment of Patients with Suicidal Behaviors* (American Psychiatric Association, 2003). Continued assessment is imperative throughout treatment, especially because the patient will experience new emotions. Learning how to tolerate and regulate these emotions may be especially difficult to accomplish.

Weight as Percentage of Healthy Body Weight As with medical status, this factor requires the lead and judgment of a physician and even also a registered dietitian if possible. The primary care physician and dietitian will discuss BMI (Body Mass Index) with the treating clinician. Generally, if body weight is less than 85% of expected, then residential treatment or inpatient hospitalization is necessary. In addition, if there is an acute weight decline with food refusal, even if the patient is not below 85% of healthy body weight, inpatient hospitalization is critical. Although tables list percentages of expected healthy body weight in relation to suggested levels of care, they are based on standardized values for the population as a whole. For any given individual, differences in body build, body composition, and other physiological variables may result in considerable differences as to what constitutes a healthy body weight in relation to "norms." Remember, when in doubt about any of these factors: CONSULT, CONSULT, and CONSULT.

Besides these three criteria, there are numerous additional factors that relate to appropriate levels of care, which are also included in the level of care guidelines (La Via et al, 1998).[46]

Motivation to Recover The more motivated a patient is, especially in terms of intrinsic versus extrinsic motivation, the more likely it is that they will respond to treatment at a lower level of care. Motivation to recover includes cooperativeness, insight, and the ability to control obsessive thoughts. The less motivated and more preoccupied one is with intrusive thoughts, the higher the level of care will be more likely indicated.

Co-occurring Disorders As stated earlier in Chapter 2, co-occurring disorders are extremely common with eating disorders. Formerly known as dual diagnoses or dual disorder, co-occurring disorders describe the presence of two or more disorders at the same time. For example, a person may suffer from bulimia as well as bipolar disorder. Some of the psychiatric disorders that can be (but are not always) found in people suffering with anorexia and bulimia are: Obsessive Compulsive Disorder, Depression, Alcohol/drug addiction, Bipolar Disorder, Post Traumatic Stress Disorder, Anxiety Disorders, Borderline Personality Disorder, Dissociative Disorder and Psychotic Disorders. Some of these disorders may influence the development of an eating disorder, and some are consequences of it. A diagnosis of co-occurring disorders is given when at least one disorder of each type can be established independently of the other, and does not represent merely a group of symptoms resulting from one disorder. Quite often, eating disorders and co-occurring disorders reinforce and "feed" one another, resulting in a vicious cycle.

Structure Needed for Eating/Gaining Weight Often the eating disorder patient requires more supervision and support eating meals. A patient may indicate that they are "eating more" when they are being seen on an outpatient basis. Remember, secrecy and manipulation are psychological factors which are clearly correlated with eating disorders. A patient may also indicate, or not, that one particular meal is more difficult to eat than another. In this case, intensive outpatient care may be a compromising alternative. At this level of care, lunch or dinner is eaten with other patients and supervised by a qualified staff member. The staff can also assist the patient in identifying and stopping food rituals, and help to reduce negative feelings and intrusive thoughts that may arise while eating.

Ability to control compulsive exercising This factor alone is rarely a sole indicator for a higher level of care.

Purging behaviors (laxatives and diuretics) If medical complications have arisen as a result of the use of these regulatory behaviors, a higher level of care may be indicated.

Environmental Stress A stable support system increases the likelihood of a stronger recovery, possibly even improving the prognosis. Attempting recovery in a high conflict environment is difficult and contributes an additional vulnerability factor that is out of the patient's control.

Geographic Availability of Treatment Program Where the patient resides may be a factor in determining the level of care they receive. A patient may live in close proximity to a treatment program or the treatment program that may best serve the patient may be too distant for them to participate in from home.

Source. Adapted and modified from La Via et al. (1998).[53] None of these guidelines is absolute, however, the application of these guidelines requires a physician's judgment.

8

THE CLINICAL INTERVIEW

The Initial Clinical Interview

Today is the first day of the rest of your life
-Anonymous

During the initial intake, the therapist gathers pertinent information. As mentioned earlier in Chapter 4, however, it is imperative that qualified specialists in various fields including a primary care physician, psychiatrist, and nutritionist see the clients.

The therapist should assess the physical, intrapersonal, interpersonal, behavioral, psychological-emotional, educational-occupational and religious-spiritual systems. More specifically, an assessment covers the following areas: Review of current problems, symptoms and reason for seeking treatment, current and past psychiatric history, history of treatment, mental status examination, medical history, family history, developmental history (e.g. development, school, work), current stressors, social support system, current and past suicidality, current and past self-harm behaviors, and other areas bases on the judgment of the evaluation team (e.g., relapse history, patterns of hospitalization. The assessment process for inpatient treatment is more extensive and involved than assessment for outpatient care.

The eating disorder history should include more specifics including current weight and the lowest and highest weight ever weighed. The complete health history should most definitely include menstrual data as well as medication history to current. It is critical to establish one's patterns and history of dieting, fasting, or avoiding to assess a potential for anorexia nervosa. This is also why it is very important to gather the information regarding current weight, highest weight, and lowest weight along with the approximate year to help correlate a connections. In order to assess for bulimia nervosa and its sub-types, the clinician must gather information about historical and current purge behaviors, such as vomiting, laxatives use, diuretic use, over the counter weight loss remedies, and excessive exercise. In addition, it is critical to assess other unhealthy weight control behaviors. As noted earlier on, examples include any behavior that is used to try to control weight or hunger, such as excessive gum-chewing, keeping clothes that are too small, going to pro-anorexia web sites, looking at photographs of models who are at very low weights, tearing food into small pieces, covering food with extra condiments, collecting cookbooks or menus, shopping, cooking, and feeding others. Food checking and ritualistic behaviors surrounding food, body checking, avoidance of body exposure, and body image concerns surrounding food must all be thoroughly assessed. In this portion of the assessment, the clinician is most often able to get a sense of any possible denial, secrecy, or minimization (e.g., "my symptoms are not bad enough to warrant this type of treatment, there are so many worse off than me) or the tendency to utilize the defense mechanism of rationalization (e.g., "I can stop anytime or I only do it when I am or have been around my family.") I have noticed that clients are often surprised at this point in the intake because suddenly many of them actually believe their secrets are no longer theirs. I have often heard, "Well how did you know that?" Sometimes this portion of the clinical assessment may also provide a sense of relief, because the patient no longer feels alone. More specific self-report assessment tools will be discussed.

Another important and often missed piece of a thorough intake is a spiritual assessment. The overall goal of a religious and spiritual assessment is to gain a clear understanding of each patient's current spiritual framework so that treatment professionals can work within the patient's belief system in a sensitive and respectful manner.[83] To find specific religious-spirituals assessments and questionnaires, refer to *Spiritual Approaches in the Treatment of Women with Eating Disorders*.[82,83] It is suggested that there are at least five reasons therapist should assess their patients' religious and spiritual backgrounds, beliefs, and lifestyle.[82,83]

(1) Conducting a religious-spiritual assessment can help therapists better understand their patients' worldviews and thus increase their capacity to empathize and work with each patient sensitively.

(2) Conducting a religious-spiritual assessment can help therapists determine whether a patient's religious-spiritual orientation is healthy or unhealthy and what impact it is having on the presenting problems and disturbance.

(3) Conducting a religious-spiritual assessment can help therapists determine whether a patient's religious and spiritual belief and community could be used as a resource to help them cope, heal, and grow.

(4) Conducting a religious-spiritual assessment can help therapists determine which spiritual interventions could be used in therapy.

(5) Conducting a religious-spiritual assessment can help therapists determine whether patients have unresolved spiritual doubts, concerns, or needs that should be addressed in therapy.

Self-Report Instruments

There are numerous psychometric assessment tools, such as interviews, surveys and questionnaires that have been developed to help professionals assess behaviors and underlying issues related to eating disorders. Self-report screening questionnaires all include questions regarding personal eating and dieting habits, weight, exercise, menstruation, body shape perception, self-image, self-esteem, drug use, relationship with the family and others, among other topics, given that most of the time patients with incipient eating disorders go to the doctor due to other symptomatology, such as weight loss, amenorrhea, depression, irritability, etc.[9] These self-report instruments were not designed to be the sole means for identifying eating disorders or to take the place of a professional diagnosis or consultation. However, they are extremely beneficial tools, especially used in conjunction with a formal interview, and can also be utilized throughout treatment to monitor progress. Here we discuss some of the more popular self-report instruments utilized

Eating Attitudes Test (EAT-26)

This is one of the most widely used screening measures that may be able to help determine if one has an eating disorder that needs professional attention. The EAT-26 has been particularly useful as a screening tool to assess "eating disorder risk" in high school, college, and other special risk groups such as athletes.[28] Designed to identify older adolescents and adults with anorexia nervosa from weight-preoccupied, but otherwise healthy female college students.

Child Eating Attitudes Test (ChEAT)

This is a version for children of the EAT-26

Eating Disorder Inventory (EDI)

One of the most widely used self-report measures, the EDI assesses the thinking patterns and behavioral characteristics of anorexia nervosa, bulimia nervosa, and eating disorders not otherwise specified (EDNOS). Ten years after the development of the original EDI, Garner published the EDI-2 as a second version the inventory. The Eating Disorder Inventory 2 (EDI-2) contains the original items from the Eating Disorder Inventory (EDI) with an additional three subscales for a total of 11 subscales. The 11 subscales include (1) drive for thinness, (2) bulimia, (3) body dissatisfaction, (4) ineffectiveness, (5) perfectionism, (6) interpersonal distrust, (7) interoceptive awareness, (8) maturity fears, (9) asceticism, (10) impulse regulation, and (11) social insecurity.[29]

Eating Disorder Examination Questionnaire (EDE-Q)

The Eating Disorder Examination Questionnaire (EDE-Q) is a self-report version of a structured interview known as the Eating Disorder Examination (EDE) designed for situations when an interview cannot be used. The EDE and EDE-Q comprises four subscales: dietary restraint, eating concern, weight concern, and shape concern.[9,23]

Revised Bulimia Test (BULIT_R)

This screens and identifies individuals who may meet the criteria for bulimia nervosa. This test assesses the behavioral, physiological, and cognitive symptoms of bulimia nervosa.[99] It contains 36 items that inquire about binge eating, purging behavior, negative affect, and weight fluctuations.

Motivation Assessments

*If you want to succeed you should strike out on new paths,
rather than travel the worn paths of accepted success.*

-*John D. Rockefeller*

Assessing readiness and barriers to change is of critical importance for successful recovery. Although the application of *readiness and motivation for change models* for the assessment and treatment of the eating disorders is still in its early stages, there is a lengthy history of work on ambivalence about change in substance abuse populations.[62] In the treatment of eating disorders, use of these motivational assessments tools would be most effective if discussion would explore all aspects of the individual's eating disorder, given that readiness and motivation for change may differ with regards to specific eating disorder symptoms. For example, one may be more willing to change one's binge eating behavior, but may express great ambivalence in decreasing one's excessive exercise routing. Both the Readiness and Motivation Interview (RMI) and the Stages of Change Model are further discussed below.

Readiness and Motivation Interview (RMI)

The RMI is a semi-structured interview designed to assess readiness and motivation for change in eating disorders. Clients are asked to talk about the extent to which they experience each relevant area as a problem. The therapist then uses follow-up questions to explore why or why not each symptom is (or is not) a problem. The therapist then prompts the client to determine how much of the client is actively working to reduce the symptom, how much of the client does not want to change the symptom at all, and how much of the client wants to change the symptom, but isn't actually doing anything change at this time.[28] The therapist also prompts the client to identify how much of the work the client is doing is intrinsically versus extrinsically motivated as well as, exploring any barriers to change. The Readiness and Motivation Interview results in a comprehensive picture of readiness and motivation for change across different areas of the eating disorder.

Stages of Change Model

The Stages of Change model shows that for most individuals, a change in behavior occurs gradually, with the patient moving from being uninterested, unaware or unwilling to make a change, to considering a change to deciding and preparing to make a change.[80] Taking action continually over time, notably with success, will most likely lead to maintenance of the new behavior. In addition, the Stages of Change Model is also beneficial to utilize with the family and significant others in order help them better understand and effectively communicate with the sufferer.

A. PRECONTEMPLATION STAGE:

> *When someone says: "Life is hard," I always ask: "Compared to what?"*
>
> -Doug Pamenter

During the pre-contemplation stage, there is no intention to change. There may be denial of a problem, a belief that the consequences are not serious enough, or a reoccurrence of unsuccessful attempts to change that they simply have given up. At this stage, it is necessary to provide education to the sufferer about the tremendous effects the eating disorder currently have or will eventually have on the individual's health and life as well as the positive aspects of change.

B. CONTEMPLATION STAGE:

*What the caterpillar calls the end, the
rest of the world calls a butterfly*

-Lao Tsu

During the contemplation stage, there is an awareness of a problem, thought about the problem, but strong ambivalence and no commitment to change. The fear of change may be very strong, and it is during this phase that a psychotherapist should assist the individual in discovering the function of the eating disorder so the individual can understand why it is part of their life and how it no longer serves any useful purpose

C. PREPARATION STAGE:

*Strength does not come from physical capacity;
it comes from an indomitable will.*

–Gandhi

During the preparation stage, there is an intention to and preparation for change, but little action is still taken. However, an individual may experiment with small changes as determination increases.

D. ACTION STAGE:

*Surrender to what is. Say, "yes" to life and see how life
suddenly starts working for your rather than against you.*

–Eckhart Tolle

During the action stage, the individual is in the process of modifying behavior, thoughts, and environment in order to overcome the problem. The individual is focused on facing personal fears, practicing flexibility, learning to identify and assert needs versus using the eating disorder to speak, engaged in meal plan compliance, being honest, and reaching out to others when she may have urges to engage in self-destructive behaviors. Overall, the individual is focused on replacing her eating disorder behaviors with recovery-based behaviors, and clearly understands what is needed for successful recovery. The individual is far more likely to move into the maintenance phase as long as that person has a strong treatment team and support system in place.

E. MAINTENANCE STAGE:

When someone tells you that you cannot go any further, just tell them to look behind you and see how far you have come.

−Lorna Pitre

During the maintenance stage, the individual is usually engaging in self-care and utilizing healthy coping skills. The person has let go of self-destructive behaviors and is focused on learning, practicing and living a life in recovery. Relapse prevention work is also of focus during this stage.

Well-phrased questions will leave the client thinking about the answers that are right for them and will move them along the process of change. *Miller WR and Rollnick S*[61] provided some examples of questions for clients in the precontemplation and contemplation stages, as seen below:

Precontemplation stage

Goal: Patient will begin thinking about change.

What would have to happen for you to know this is a problem?

What warning signs would let you know that this is a problem?

Have you tried to change in the past?

Contemplation stage

Goal: Patient will examine benefits and barriers to change.

Why do you want to change at this time?

What were the reasons for not changing?

What would keep you from changing at this time?

What are the barriers today that keep you from change?

What might help you with that aspect?

What things (people, programs and behaviors) have helped you in the past?

What would help you at this time?

The individual may need to revisit particular stages when focusing on specific symptoms of the eating disorder. For example, the individual may be in the Action stage in regards to meal plan compliance, yet still in the Pre-contemplation stage with the symptom of over-exercising. Alternatively, the individual may be in the Preparation stage in regards to reaching out to others and utilizing her support system to avoid isolation. At the same time, the individual may be going through the Contemplation stage with the symptom of comparing the self to others. Recovery from an eating disorder is unique to each individual. Remember, there is no perfection in recovery.

Additional Patient Assessment Tools

As previously discussed, there is a strong association between eating disorders and depression, anxiety, and obsessive-compulsive disorder. The Becks scales and inventories are validated tools to assist in measuring the severity of depressive and anxiety symptoms. These inventories may also be utilized in conjunction with the eating disorder self-report instruments and may also be very beneficial to utilize throughout treatment.

Beck Anxiety Inventory (BAI)

The Beck Anxiety Inventory (BAI) is a 21-item scale, rated on a 4-point scale, which measures the severity of self-reported anxiety symptoms in adults and adolescents. The Beck Anxiety Inventory was specifically designed to reduce the overlap between depression and anxiety scales by measuring anxiety symptoms shared minimally with those of depression.[6]

Beck Depression Inventory (BDI-II)

This new revised edition replaces the original Beck Depression Inventory (BDI) and now indicates increases or decreases in sleep and appetite, items labeled body image, work difficulty, and weight loss.[7,8] The Beck Depression Inventory Second Edition (BDI-II) is a 21-item self-report intended to identify the presence and severity of depressive symptoms consistent with the criteria in the American Psychiatric Association's Diagnostic and Statistical Manual of Mental Disorders Fourth Edition.[3]

Clark-Beck Obsessive-Compulsive Inventory (CBOCI)

This self-report measure of obsessive-compulsive symptoms is patterned after the BDI-II, with a similar response format and structure. It includes 11 items that assess obsessive behaviors and 14 items that assess compulsive behaviors.

Dissociative Experiences Scale (DES)

This screening test for Dissociative Identity Disorder consists of twenty-eight questions.

Integrating the results of many of these various assessments will assist in developing the most effective treatment plan for each unique individual.

9

REVISITING VIGNETTES IN RECOVERY

Freedom and Life after an Eating Disorder

"You've gotta dance like there's nobody watching,
Love like you'll never be hurt,
Sing like there's nobody listening,
And live like it's heaven on earth."

-William W. Purkey

Remember Laura: *When Laura was 18, she went away to college. She made friends, went to her classes, and went to parties with her peers. Laura was living in the dorm with several other girls. She found herself continually comparing herself to all of them. Watching them undress, she eyed their "skinny and perfect bodies" and thought "why can't I be like that?" Laura listened to them talk about a new diet every week and participated in every new trend, but no matter how hard she tried, Laura "never" felt enough next to all of these other girls. Thoughts like these began to consume her. These were not new thoughts or feelings, but they had never been so intense. This being Laura's first time away from home, she thought that the freedom was going to be incredible. She did not anticipate the response she was experiencing, how lonely she would actually feel or the competitiveness that would consume her.*

But one day, Laura came home from class early only to find candy wrappers, a pizza box, and an empty pint on ice cream sitting on her bed. Next, she heard someone gagging in the bathroom and Laura immediately knew what she was up too. Laura quickly left the room, as she wanted to avoid any confrontation with her roommate. The thoughts raced through her mind; "now I know how she stays so thin. I can do that and I can eat more. I don't have to do these stupid diets anymore. Maybe I have finally found the cure. I can eat whatever I want, lose weight, and feel better. My life can get better and I will finally feel like I fit in and life can be good, really good." This was the beginning of the binge-purge cycle that would ultimately bring Laura to the lowest point she ever experienced in her lifetime.

In the beginning, it felt like Laura's dreams were coming true. Laura had a secret. She believed she had it all under control and had found the answer to happiness. She could eat whatever she wanted, and she did, and she could vomit it all away after. Laura began to spend the majority of her money on food. Laura would consume her food so quickly and eat until she felt so full and so sick that all she wanted to do was go to sleep. That was not an option until she vomited and there was nothing left to come up. Throwing up became easier and easier but increasingly difficult to hide. The desperation set it and Laura would vomit into plastic bags and cups, at times not throwing them away for days at a time.

Yet, as quickly as she believed she had found the answer, everything fell apart and Laura found that every part of her life was affected. Laura became completely preoccupied with thoughts of food, weight, and appearance. Her bingeing and purging became her best friend and her worst enemy.

Laura's friendships became distant and even more shallow, her grades began to drop, she became short tempered with her parents each time she spoke with them on the phone, and she began to have constant headaches and sore throats. To make matters worse, Laura was not even losing weight. "Wasn't this why I started this in the first place?" Things that were of value and importance to Laura suddenly didn't seem to matter anymore. The shame and guilt lead Laura into feeling more despair and anxiety. All of these factors only fueled that cycle. Only one thing seemed to quiet her head and so she thought made her feel better, well at least for a moment, and that was bingeing and purging.

LAURA IN RECOVERY

Laura did finally break her silence by reaching out to health services on her college campus. She did leave school for a period of time to receive the treatment she needed. Laura was initially treated in an inpatient facility to become medically stabilized. From there, she stepped down to lower levels of care. The first step down was to a day treatment program, next to an individualized outpatient program, and finally to an outpatient level of care. Laura did get her life back. Laura is mindful and vigilant on a daily basis. Before she returned to school she had a treatment team consisting of a therapist, a nutritionist, psychiatrist, and a primary care physician. She also had referrals to other professionals who are trained to work with eating disorders. These included a dentist to continue to assist her with the damage she had done to her teeth, a gastroenterologist (GI) for any digestive problems that may need to be treated, as well as a gynecologist for optimal management of reproductive issues. With the help of the treatment center, Laura was able to make sure that all the primary practitioners had releases signed to communicate with one another. In addition, Laura attends a support group on the school campus as well as attending various 12-step meetings such as Overeater's Anonymous (OA) and Eating Disorders Anonymous (EDA). Laura also goes to yoga to learn how to become more mindful and connected to her body. She clearly understands that recovery requires a community. In addition, Laura's family became educated and participated in the family treatment offered at the treatment center. They too continue to receive the support they need to work on their issues or concerns and learn how to help Laura the best way possible. At times, she does still struggle with thoughts about weight, food, and body, and even finds herself comparing to others. The difference is that Laura has a high motivation and readiness for change. She has the tools to challenge and replace those thoughts and understands the importance of emotional regulation. She has learned that recovery takes place on so many levels: intrapersonal (within oneself), interpersonal (relationships), cognitive (thoughts), emotional (regulation of emotions), occupational, and spiritual (faith, love, gratitude, honesty and compassion).

Remember Rachel, *a 32 year old female, reported her first significant weight loss during her first year of college away from home. She had been in numerous treatment centers since that time and reports that recovery has been an ongoing struggle. Rachel had always been very athletic as a young girl. This included being a dancer as well as avid runner. She had consistently been a good student and had placed very high expectations of herself from as long as she could remember. She has an incredible fear of being "fat" and will do whatever is need to this at all costs. Rachel dressed in baggy clothes, wearing several layers, and describes her reasoning as being cold all of the time.*

In regards to an example of an average day with food and exercise, Rachel wakes up by 5:00 am, but on the weekend she allows herself to sleep until 5:30 am. She begins her day with a large cup of coffee from the same large cup she uses daily. She pours a splash of fat free creamer and uses 3 packets of an alternative sweetener along with one teaspoon of honey, but she insists that it must be one particular brand. Rachel then puts on her running shoes, rain or shine, and runs for 1.5 hours. Upon return, Rachel takes off her clothes and immediately steps on the scale. This will be her determining factor for the entire rest of her day, including her mood and her food intake. After she scrutinizes her body by touching her bones, measuring her wrist size, she proceeds to eat breakfast. This either consists of a 4 oz. bowl of oatmeal with several packets of an alternative sweetener along with a quarter cup of nonfat milk or a container of vanilla nonfat yogurt with 10 blueberries. Breakfast is followed by another weigh in and body check before she proceeds to shower and get ready for her day. Rachel sticks a rigid regime of no more than 750 calories a day. She only allows herself to eat specific foods at the same time every day. Her food choices have become increasingly limited over the many years she has struggled with anorexia.

RACHEL IN RECOVERY

We begin with Rachel and her physical recovery, which is assessed by weight restoration, return of menses, and management of medical complications. Following several hospitalizations and continual intervention by Rachel's family and closest friend, she made a decision to enter treatment again. Her initial treatment goal of weight restoration took place in an inpatient treatment setting. Early treatment focused on identifying, stabilizing and treating medical complications. Once there was an increase in her Body Mass Index (BMI or percentile of ideal body weight), her menses returned. Rachel then stepped down to a partial hospitalization program followed by an individualized outpatient program to transition back into her life. She was diagnosed with osteopernia and is currently being treated by her primary care physician and a rheumatologist. In addition, Rachel was prescribed medication for anxiety by the psychiatrist.

Rachel has continued in outpatient treatment with a treatment team in place. Her motivation for change shifted as she was faced with letting go of specific eating disorder behaviors, as some were more of a challenge than others. Rachel's early treatment also included psychoeducation, dietary change, and cognitive restructuring, to address core beliefs (e.g., "My weight will go out of control if I do not restrict." "If I eat normally, I will start to binge?"). Her cognitive functioning improved with weight restoration resulting in an increased ability to engage in more insight-oriented treatment. The therapist continued to utilize CBT to reduce the ritualistic behaviors and to challenge her cognitive distortions. In addition to the cognitive behavior treatment modality, Rachel has responded exceptionally well to Dialectical Behavioral Therapy, also known as DBT. DBT focuses on mindfulness, distress tolerance, emotional regulation, and interpersonal effectiveness. Putting all of these skills into practice has been an integral part of her recovery.

Rachel has continued to work with the dietitian and has followed a meal plan far beyond her discharge from her last hospitalization, as there is no recovery without weight gain. Weight maintenance is now an ongoing goal. Learning to integrate these skills into daily life is something that Rachel and the nutritionist continually work with. Rachel is learning how to cook, shop at the market, prepare her food, and increase her comfort level to be able to eat with others. Exercise goals have shifted throughout treatment. Due to the disconnect that Rachel has experienced through her years struggling with an eating disorder, she has integrated other therapies to help her reconnect to her body and her overall femininity. And with much exploration and support from others, including her gynecologist, Rachel has come to a place of acceptance with a decision to not have children. She has gained awareness and appreciation of herself through yoga, meditation, women's retreats, and practicing mindfulness when walking and hiking. Rachel also found that Overeater's Anonymous was not an appropriate match, but she connected instead to Eating Disorder's Anonymous. Rachel has learned how to allow room for mistakes, continually practicing loving kindness and patience with herself. Rachel did eventually return to school, but with a completely new intention, to become a nutritionist. She found a job that emphasizes her strengths, but differently than she used them in her eating disorder. For example, throughout her eating disorder she was orderly and a perfectionist. Now, she uses these traits to help her maintain strong organizational skills. She is extremely reliable. Rachel has learned how to live again.

Not everyone is so lucky to enter a life of recovery. There are far too many who do not win their battle with these deadly disorders. Hence, our knowledge may just save a life.

Epilogue: Last Words

Eating disorders are dangerous, all encompassing, and can ultimately result in tragedy. If you know anyone who may be suffering from any of these eating disorders or believe that you are witnessing warning signs, please intervene. WE must continue to work at all levels to become educated and learn to walk on a MINDFULPATH of recovery. WE need to teach the public about these tragic eating disorders that are afflicting our youth, digging deeper into our adolescents, and immersing themselves into our adults. WE can no longer allow the secrecy that surrounds eating disorders to keep us silent or in the dark. WE must continue to gain more insight and knowledge into the world of eating disorders, and just as we let the sufferers know that they are not alone, you too are not alone in fighting the battle of eating disorders.

About the Author

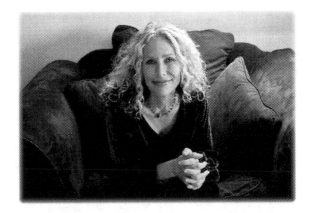

Erica Ives, M.A., MFT, CEDS is a certified eating disorder specialist and the owner of Mindfulpath, Inc. A graduate from Pepperdine University, Erica has been practicing as a Marriage and Family Therapist for nearly twenty years. Her own personal struggles led to her passionate devotion to this field of healing. Her work as a therapist began with the treatment of adolescents who struggled with drug and alcohol addiction, eating disorders, self-injury and various other self-destructive behaviors predominately as a result of some form of trauma. She sought out extensive training in the area of trauma and its correlation with the development of all types of addiction. Her many years of training and experience developed into her current area of specialization.

She has maintained a private practice in Calabasas while simultaneously working closely with other professionals and clients in a multiple array of environments. She has worked as a Clinical Director, as a CAMFT Certified Clinical Supervisor, and as a consultant for several treatment centers. She has educated communities on prevention, the treatment of eating disorders and substance abuse, and she has published numerous articles on these topics. Erica whole-heartedly believes in life with freedom from eating disorders and all types of addiction. She views recovery as being unique to each individual and she teaches the tools for achieving a life filled with balance, awareness, and an overall sense of well being. For more information, visit her websites at www. mindfulpath.com and www.ericaives.com.

References

1. Alcoholics Anonymous. *Alcoholics Anonymous, The Big Book*. New York: Alcoholics Anonymous World Services, 1995.

2. American Dietetic Association. Position of the American Dietetic Association: Nutrition intervention in the treatment of eating disorders. *J Am Diet Association*. 2011; 111:1236-1241.

3. American Psychiatric Association (2000): *Diagnostic and Statistical Manual of Mental Disorders (4th ed. Text Revision)*. Washington, DC: American Psychiatric Association.

4. American Psychiatric Association. (2000). Practice guidelines for the treatment of patients with eating disorders (revision). *American Journal of Psychiatry, 157*, 1-39.

5. American Psychiatric Association. *Practice Guideline for the Treatment of Patients with Eating Disorders*, Third Edition, June 2006.

6. Beck, Aaron T. and Robert A. Steer. *Beck Anxiety Inventory Manual*. San Antonio, TX: The Psychological Corporation Harcourt Brace & Company, 1993.

7. Beck A.T, Ward C.H., Mendelson, J. Mock, and Erbaugh. "An inventory for measuring depression. *Arch Gen Psychiatry* 4 (1961): 561-571.

8. Beck A.T., and R. A. Steer. "Internal consistencies of the original and revised Beck Depression Inventory." *Journal of Clinical Psychology*. 40.1 (November 1984): 1365-7.

9. Black, C. M., Wilson, G. T. "Assessment of eating disorders: interview or self-report questionnaire?" *International Journal of Eating Disorders* 20 (1996): 43-50.

10. Bograd, M., "Enmeshment: Fusion or Relatedness: A Conceptual Analysis." *Journal of Psychotherapy and the Family*, 3, 4: 65-80.

11. Brewerton, T. "Eating Disorders, Trauma, and Comorbity: Focus on PTSD." *Eating Disorders*, 15 (2007): 285-304.

12. Bulik, C.M. "Exploring the Gene-environment Nexus in Eating Disorders." *Journal of Psychiatry & Neuroscience*, 30 (2005): 335-339.

13. Bulik, C. M., P. F. Sullivan, and K. S. Kendler. "Heritability of binge-eating and broadly defined bulimia nervosa. *Biol Psychiatry* 44 (1998): 1210-1218.

14. Bulik, C.M., P. F. Sullivan, and K. S. Kendler. "Twin studies of eating disorders: a review." *International Journal of Eating Disorders* 27 (2000): 1-20.

15. Clinical Practice Guideline for Eating Disorders. Madrid: Quality Plan for the National Health System of the Ministry of Health and Consumer Affairs. Catalan Agency for Health Technology Assessment and Research; 2009. Clinical Practice Guidelines in the NHS: CAHTA Number 2006/05-01.

16. Crowther, J. H., E. M. Wolf, and N. Sherwood. "Epidemiology of bulimia nervosa." *The Etiology of Bulimia Nervosa: The Individual and Familial Context*. Eds. M. Crowther, D. L. Tennenbaum, S. E. Hobfoll, and M. A. P. Stephens. Washington, D.C.: Taylor & Francis, 1992. 1-16.

17. Davis, R., and M. Olmsted, M. "Cognitive-behavioral group treatment for bulimia nervosa: Integrating psychoeducation and psychotherapy." *Group Psychotherapy for eating disorders*. Eds. H. Harper-Giuffre and K. R. MacKenzie. Washington, DC: American Psychiatric Press, 1992.

18. Day, Jemma, et al. "Risk Factors, Correlates, and Markers in Early-Onset Bulimia Nervosa and EDNOS." *Int. J Eat Disord* 44 (2011): 287-294.

19. Deep, A. L., L. R. Lilenfeld, K. H. Plotnicov, C. Pollice, and W. H. Kaye. "Sexual abuse in eating disorder subtypes and control women: The role of comorbid substance dependence in bulimia nervosa." *The International Journal of Eating Disorders*, 25 (1999): 1-10.

20. Ellison A.R., and J. Fong. "Neuroimaging in eating disorders." *Neurobiology in the Treatment of Eating Disorders*. Eds. H. W. Hoek, J. L. Treasure, and M. A. Katzman. Chichester: Wiley, 1998. 255-269.

21. Fairburn, C. G., P. J. Hay, and S. L. Welch. "Binge eating and bulimia nervosa: Distribution and determinants." *Binge Eating: Nature, Assessment, and Treatment*. Eds. C. G. Fairburn and G. T. Wilson. New York: Guilford, 1993. 123-143.

22. Fairburn, C. G. *Overcoming Binge Eating.* New York, NY: Guilford Press, 1995.

23. Fairburn, C. G., and Z. Cooper. The Eating Disorder Examination. (12th ed.) In C.G. Fairburn, & G.T. Wilson (Eds.) *Binge Eating: Nature, Assessment, and Treatment.* New York: Guilford Press, (1993.) 317-360.

24. Fairburn, C. G., and S. J. Beglin. "Assessment of eating disorder psychopathology: interview or self-report questionnaire?" *International Journal of Eating Disorders* 16 (1994). 363-370.

25. Field, A. E., K. M. Javaras, P. Angela, N. Kitos, C. A. Camargo, J., C. B. Taylor, et al. "Family, peer, and media predictors of becoming eating disordered." *Arch Pediatric Adolescent Med.* 162.6 (June 2008): 574-9.

26. Fox, J. R. E., and A. Harrison. "The relationship of anger to disgust: The potential role of coupled emotions within eating pathology." *Clinical Psychology and Psychotherapy,* 15 (2008):86-95.

27. Garner D.M. Omsted, M.P., Bohr, Y. and Garfinkel, P.E., "The Eating Attitudes Test: Psychometric features and clinical correlates." *Psychological Medicine, 12,* (1982): 871-878.

28. Garner, D. M., and M. P. Olmsted. The Eating Disorder Inventory Manual. Odessa, FL: *Psychological Assessment Resources,* 1983

29. Garner, D. M. Eating Disorder Inventory-2 Professional Manual. Odessa, FL: Psychological Assessment Resources, 1991.

30. Geller J., and D. Drab. "The Readiness and Motivation Interview: A symptom-specific measure of readiness for change in the eating disorders." *European Eat Discord Rev 7* (1999): 259-278.

31. Geller J., S. L. Zaitsoff, and S. J. Cockell. Clinical Decision-Making: Contribution of Readiness and Motivation Information. Paper presented at the meeting of the Eating Disorders Research Society, Bavria, Germany, 2000.

32. Gidwani, G.P., and E.S. Rome. Eating Disorders. *Clinical Obstetrics and Gynecology* 40.3 (1997): 601-615.

33. Gilligan C., A. G. Rogers, and D. L. Tolman. *Women, Girls and Psychotherapy: Reframing Resistance.* The Haworth Press, Inc., Binghamton, NY, 1991.

34. Gleaves D.H., D. A. Williamson, and S. E. "Addictive effects of mood and eating forbidden foods upon the perceptions of overeating and binging in bulimia nervosa." *Addict Behav* 18 (1993): 299-305.

35. Goodman, S., H. G. Slotnick, W. J. Swift, and S. A. Wonderlich. "DSM-III-R Personality Disorders in Eating-Disorder Subtypes." *International Journal of Eating Disorders,* 9 (2006): 607-616.

36. Gordon, R.A. *Anorexia and Bulimia: Anatomy of a Social Epidemic.* New York: Blackwell, 1990.

37. Graber, J.A., and J. Brooks-Gunn. "Growing up female: Navigating body image, eating, and depression." *Journal of Emotional and Behavioral Problems,* 5.2 (1996): 76-80.

38. Halmi, K. A. "Eating Disorders: Anorexia nervosa, bulimia nervosa, and obesity."*APP Textbook of psychiatry.* Eds. R. E. Hales, S. C. Yudofsky, and J. A. Talbott. Washington, DC: American Psychiatric Press, (1994). 857-876.

39. Harper-Giuffre, H., and K. R. MacKenzie. "Interpersonal Group Psychotherapy." *Group Psychotherapy for eating disorders.* Eds. H. Harper-Giuffre and K. R. MacKenzie. Washington, DC: American Psychiatric Press, 1992.

40. Haworth-Hoeppner, S. "The critical shapes of body image: The role of culture and family in the production of eating disorders." *Journal of Marriage and Family* 62.1 (2000): 212-227.

41. Hendrix, H. Getting the love you want. New York, NY: Holt & Company, 1998.

42. Hoek, H. W. "The distribution of eating disorders." *Eating Disorders and Obesity: A Comprehensive Handbook.* Eds. K. D. Brownell and C. G. Fairburn. New York: Guilford, 1995. 207-211.

43. Hoek, H. W., and D. van Hoeken, D. "Review of the prevalence and incidence of eating disorders." *International Journal of Eating Disorders* (2003): 383-396.

44. Hudson, J.I., Hiripi, E., Pope, H. G., and R. C.Kessler. "The Prevalence and Correlate of Eating Disorders in the National Comorbidity Survey Replication," *Biol Psychiatry* 61(3), (2007): 348-358.

45. Insel, T.R., M.D., Director of the National Institute of Mental Health, October 5, 2006.

46. Johnson, C. L., and R. A. Samsone. "Integrating the 12-step approach with traditional psychotherapy for the treatment of eating disorders." *International Journal of Eating Disorders* 14 (1993): 121-134.

47. Kaplan, A. S., and P. E. Garfinkel. *Medical issues and the eating disorders: The interface.* New York: Brunner/Mazel, 1993.

48. Kaplan, H. I., and B. J. Sadock. *Synopsis of psychiatry* (8thed.). Baltimore, MD: Williams and Wilkens, 1998.

49. Kaye, W, A. Wagner, and G. Frank, Uf B. "Review of brain imaging in anorexia and bulimia nervosa." *AED Annual Review of Eating Disorders, Part 2*. Eds. J. Mitchell, S.Wonderlich, H. Steiger, and M. Dezwaan. Abingdon, UK: Radcliffe Publishing Ltd, 2006. 113-130.

50. Kendler K.S., M. C. Neale, et al. "Generalized anxiety disorder in women. A population-based twin study." *Archives of General Psychiatry* 49.4 (1992): 267-72.

51. Kerr, M., and Bowen, M., 1988. Family Evaluation: An Approach Based on Bowen Theory, NY, Norton.

52. Kessler, R.C., W. T. Chiu, O. Demler, and E. E. Walters. "Prevalence, severity, and comorbidity of twelve-month DSM-IV disorders in the National Comorbidity Survey Replication (NCS-R)." *Archives of General Psychiatry* 62.6 (June 2005): 617-627.

53. La Via, M., W. H. Kaye, et al. "Anorexia nervosa: criteria for levels of care." Annual Meeting of the Eating Disorders Research Society. Cambridge, Mass, 5-7 November 1998. Paper.

54. Le Grange, D., and J. Lock. "Family-based Treatment of Adolescent Anorexia Nervosa." *The Maudsley Approach*. <http:// www.maudsleyparents.org>

55. Lesserman, J. "Sexual abuse history; Prevalence health effects, mediators, and psychological treatment." *Psychosomatic Medicine*, 67 (2005): 906-915.

56. Levine, M. (1994). "A Short List of Salient Warning Signs for Eating Disorders." 13th National NEDO Conference, Columbus, Ohio (October 3, 1994).

57. Linehan, M. M. *Cognitive-Behavioral Treatment of Borderline Personality Disorder.* New York: Guilford Press, 1993.

58. Linehan, M. M. *Skills Training Manual for Treating Borderline Personality Disorder.* New York: The Guilford Press, 1993.

59. Mehler, P. S., and A. E. Andersen, eds. *Eating disorders: A guide to medical care and complications.* Baltimore: John Hopkins University Press, 1999.

60. Mehler, P., MD. "Medical Complications of Bulimia Nervosa and their Treatments." *International Journal of Eating Disorders* 44 (2011): 95-104.

61. Miller, W.R., and S. Rollnick. *Motivational interviewing: Preparing people to change addictive behavior.* New York: Guilford Press, 1991. 191-202.

62. Miller, W.R., and S. Rollnick. Motivational interviewing: Preparing people for change. New York: Guilford Press, 1999.

63. Minuchin, S., 1974. *Families & Family Therapy*, Cambridge, MA, Harvard University Press.

64. Mitchell, K. S., S. E. Mazzeo, M. R. Schlesinger, T. D. Brewerton, and B. N. Smith. "Comorbidity of Partial and Subthreshold PTSD among Men and Women with Eating Disorders in the National Comorbidity Survey-Replication Study." *Int J Eat Disord* 45 (2012): 307-315.

65. Mitchell, J.E., and C. Pomeroy. "Medical Complications of anorexia nervosa and bulimia nervosa." *Eating Disorders and Obesity: A Comprehensive Handbook (Second Edition)*. Eds. C. G. Fairburn and K. D. Brownell. New York, New York: Guilford Press, 2001

66. Mitchell, J., and Wonderlich, S. "The role of personality in the onset of eating disorders and treatment implication." *Psychiatric Clinics of North America* 24 (2001): 249-250.

67. Mitchell, J.E., H. C. Seim, P. Colon, and P. Pomeroy. "Medical complications and medical management of bulimia." *Ann Intern Med* 107 (1987):71-76.

68. National Center for Complementary and Alternative Medicine (NCCAM). www.nccam.nih.gov

69. National Institute of Mental Health (NIMH). www.nimh.nih.gov

70. Neumark-Sztainer, D. *I'm, Like, SO Fat!* New York: Guilford, 2005.

71. Oberndorfer, T., W. Kaye, A. Simmons, I. Strigo, S. Matthews. "Demand-Specific Alteration of Medial Prefrontal Cortex Response During an Inhibition Task in Recovered Anorexic Women." *International Journal of Eating Disorders* 44 (2011): 1-8.

72. O'Brien, K., and N. Vincent. "Psychiatric comorbidity in anorexia and bulimia nervosa: Nature, prevalence, and casual relationships." *Clinical Psychology Review* 23 (2003): 57-74.

73. Office of Applied Studies. *Overview of findings from the 2002 National Survey on Drug Use and Health* (DHHS Pub. No. (SMA) 03-3774). Rockville, MD: U.S. Department of Health and Human Services, Substance Abuse and Mental Health Services Administration, Office of Applied Studies.

74. *Just for Today*. Los Angeles: Overeaters Anonymous, 1979.

75. *Questions & Answers About Compulsive Overeating and OA Program of Recovery*. Los Angeles: Overeaters Anonymous, 1979.

76. Peterson, C. B., and J. E. Mitchell. "Self-report measures." *Assessment of eating disorders*. Eds. J. E. Mitchell and C. B. Peterson. New York: Guilford Press, 2005.

77. Petitpas, A and Chanmpagne, D. *Journal of College Student Development"* 1988, 29:454-460.

78. Phillips KA. "Body dysmorphic disorder: the distress of imagined ugliness." *Am J Psychiatry* 148 (1991): 1138-1149.

79. Phillips, K. A. "Body dysmorphic disorder." *Somatoform and factitious disorders.* In: Phillips KA, editor. Ed. Washington: American Psychiatric Publishing, 2001.

80. Prochaska, J.O., C. C. DiClemente, and J. C. Norcross. "In search of how people change." *American Psychology* 47 (1992): 1101-1104.

81. Rich, A. *On lies, secrets, and silence.* New York: Norton, 1979. 188.

82. Richards, P. S., and A. E. Bergin. *A spiritual strategy for counseling and psychotherapy (2nd ed.).* Washington, DC: American Psychological Association, 2005.

83. Richards, S. P., R. K. Hardman, and M. E. Berrett. *Spiritual Approaches in the Treatment of Women With Eating Disorders.* Washington, DC: American Psychological Association, 2007.

84. Roberts, D., and U. Foehr. *Kids and Media in America.* Cambridge, MA: University Press, 2004.

85. Rosaldo, M.Z., and L. Lamphere. *Women, Culture & Society*: Stanford, Stanford University Press, 1993.

86. Roy, Praveen K., M.D., and Julian Katz, MD. "Boerhaave Syndrome." *WebMD LLC*, 18 August 2011. <http://emedicine.medscape.com/article/171683-overview>

87. Rushing, I., L. E. Jones, and C. Carney. "Bulimia Nervosa: A Primary Care Review." *Primary Care Companion J Clinical Psychiatry* 5 (2003): 217-224.

88. Samsone, R. A., and L. A. Samsone. "Personality Disorders as Risk Factors for Eating Disorders: Clinical Implications." *Nutrition in Clinical Practice.* 25 (April 2010): 116-121.

89. Schlundt, D. G., and W. G. Johnson. *Eating Disorders: Assessment and treatment.* Boston: Allyn and Bacon, 1990.

90. Schmidt, U., S. Lee, J. Beecham, et al. "A randomized controlled trial of family therapy and cognitive behavior therapy guided self-care for adolescents with bulimia nervosa and related disorders." *Am J Psychiatry.* 164.4 (Apr 2007): 591-598.

91. Shisslak, C. M., M. Crago, and L. S. Estes. "The Spectrum of eating disturbances." *International Journal of Eating Disorders* 18(3) (1995): 209-219.

92. Silverstone, P. H. "Is chronic low self-esteem the cause of eating disorders?" *Medical Hypotheses*, 39.4 (1992):311-315.

93. Smith, E. E., M. D. Marcus, C. E. Lewis, M. Fitzgibbon, and P. Schreiner. Prevalence of binge eating disorder, obesity and depression in a biracial cohort of young adults. *Annals of Behavioral Medicine*, 20 (1998): 227-232.

94. Smolak, L. *National Eating Disorders Association/Next Door Neighbors Puppet Guide Book.* 1996.

95. Steiner-Adair, C. "When the Body Speaks: Girls Eating Disorders and Psychotherapy" *Women, Girls & Psychotherapy: Reframing Resistance.* Eds. C. Gilligan, A. Rogers, and D. Tolman. New York: Haworth Press, 1991.

96. Strumia, R. "Dermatologic signs in patients with eating disorders." *Am Journal of Clinical Dermatology* 6 (2005): 165-173.

97. Sullivan, P. F. "Mortality in anorexia nervosa." *American Journal of Psychiatry.* 152.7 (1995): 1073-1074.

98. Tchanturia. K., M. B. Anderluch, R. G. Morris, S. Rabe-Hesketh, D. A. Collier, P. Sanchez et al. "Cognitive flexibility in anorexia nervosa and bulimia nervosa." *J Int Neuropsychological Soc* 10 (2004): 513-520.

99. Thelen, M. H., L. B. Mintz, and J. S. Vander Wal. "The Bulimia Test-Revised: Validation with DSM-IV criteria for bulimia nervosa." *Psychological Assessment*, 8 (1996): 219-221.

100. The National Center on Addiction and Substance Abuse at Columbia University *Food For Thought: Substance abuse and eating disorders.* New York: The National Center of Addiction and Substance Abuse at Columbia University, 2003.

101. The National Eating Disorders Association (NEDA). www.NationalEatingDisorders.org

102. Touyz, S.W., V. P. Liew, P. Tseng, K. Frisken, H. Williams, and P. J. Beumont "Oral and dental complications in eating disorders." *International Journal of Eating Disorders* 14 (1993): 341-347.

103. Von Ranson, K. M., W. G. Iacono, and M. McGue. Disordered eating and substance use in an epidemiological sample: 1. Associations within individuals. *International Journal of Eating Disorders* 31 (2002): 389-403.

104. Williams, P.M., J. Goodie, C. D. Motsinger. Treating eating disorders in primary care. *Am Fam Physician* 77.2 (January 15 2008): 187-95.

105. Yager, J, M. J. Devlin, K. A. Halmi, et al. *Practice Guidelines for the Treatment of Patients with Eating Disorders (3rd ed.)*. Washington, DC: American Psychiatric Association, 2006.

106. Yalom, I. D. *The Theory and Practice of Group Psychotherapy: 5th edition.* New York, NY: Basic Books, 2005.

107. Zerbe, K. J. *The Body Betrayed*. Carlsbad, CA: Gurze Books, 1995.

Resources

The Academy for Eating Disorders (AED)

www.aedweb.org

AED is an international professional organization that promotes research, treatment, and prevention of all types of eating disorders.

National Eating Disorders Association (NEDA)

www.NationalEatingDisorders.org

The National Eating Disorders Association is a non-profit organization dedicated to supporting individuals and families affected by eating disorders, and serves as a catalyst for prevention, cures, and access to quality care.

The National Association of Anorexia Nervosa and Associated Disorders (ANAD)

www.anad.org

The oldest national nonprofit organization dedicated to alleviating the problems of eating disorders and promoting healthy lifestyles.

International Association of Eating Disorder Professionals (IAEDP)

www.iaedp.com

Established in 1985, the International Association of Eating Disorder Professionals (IAEDP) is today well recognized for its excellence in providing first-quality education and high-level training standards to an international multidisciplinary group of various healthcare treatment providers and helping profession, who treat the full spectrum of Eating Disorder problems.

Eating Disorder Anonymous (EDA)

www.eatingdisorderanonymous.org

EDA provides information about local support group meetings and additional resources regarding eating disorders.

Gurze Books

www.gurze.com

www.bulimia.com

Publishes and distributes a wide variety of books, videos, and periodicals about eating disorders and related therapies, as well as treatment referrals.

Something Fishy

www.something-fishy.org

Dedicated to raising awareness and providing support to those suffering from an eating disorder and the loved ones who are also so greatly affected by this disorder.

National Institute of Mental Health (NIMH)

www.nimh.nih.gov

The mission of NIMH is to transform the understanding and treatment of mental illnesses through basic and clinical research, paving the way for prevention, recovery, and cure.

The National Center on Addiction and Substance Abuse at Columbia University (CASA)

www.casacolumbia.org

The National Center on Addiction and Substance Abuse at Columbia University is a science-based, multidisciplinary organization focused on transforming society's understanding of and responses to substance use and the disease of addiction.

Mirror-Mirror Website on Eating Disorders

www.mirror-mirror.org/eatdis.htm

An organization dedicated to raising awareness and providing information about eating disorders- definitions, signs and symptoms, getting help, relapse warning signs, approaching a loved one and more.

Andrea's Voice Foundation

www.andreasvoice.org

Started after the death of Andrea Smeltzer by her parents to raise awareness and promote prevention.

Eating Disorder Referral and Information Center

www.edreferral.com

The Eating Disorder Referral and Information Center provides information and treatment resources for all forms of eating disorders. This website will assist you in finding a treatment center or private practitioner specializing in eating disorders anywhere in the United States or internationally.

BodyPositive.com

Provides information and resources (including links to other websites) to promote a positive body image in people of all ages.

EAT-26 Self-Test

www.eat-26.com

The EAT-26 is the most widely used screening measure that may be able to help you determine if you have an eating disorder that needs professional attention. At this website, you can learn more about the test, download a copy, as well as find instructions regarding how to score and interpret the test.

Pearson Assessment and Information

www.pearsonassessments.com

Find clinical assessment products for better insights, better decisions, and better outcomes.

Organizations

Academy for Eating Disorders (AED)
111 Deer Lake Road, Suite 100
Deerfield, IL 60015
Phone: (847) 498-4274
aedweb.org

Eating Disorders Coalition (EDC)
720 7th Street NW, Suite 300
Washington, DC 20001
Phone: (202) 543-9570
Eatingdisorderscoalition.org

International Association of Eating Disorder Professionals (IAEDP)
PO Box 1295
Pekin, IL 61555-1295
Phone: (800) 800-8126
Iaedp.com

National Association of Anorexia Nervosa and Associated Disorders (ANAD)
750 E Diehl Road #127
Naperville, IL 60563
Phone: (630) 577-1330
anad.org

National Eating Disorders Association (NEDA)
165 West 46th Street
New York, NY 10036
Phone: (212) 575-6200
Treatment referral: (800) 931-2237
Nationaleatingdisorders.org

National Eating Disorder Information Centre (NEDIC)
ES 7-421, 200 Elizabeth Street
Toronto, Ontario M5G 2C4
Phone: (416) 340-4156
Toll-Free 1-866-NEDIC-20
Nedic.ca

Overeaters Anonymous (OA)
World Services Offices
P.O. Box 44020
Rio Rancho, NM 87124
Phone: (505) 891-2664
Oa.org

Index

D

E

M